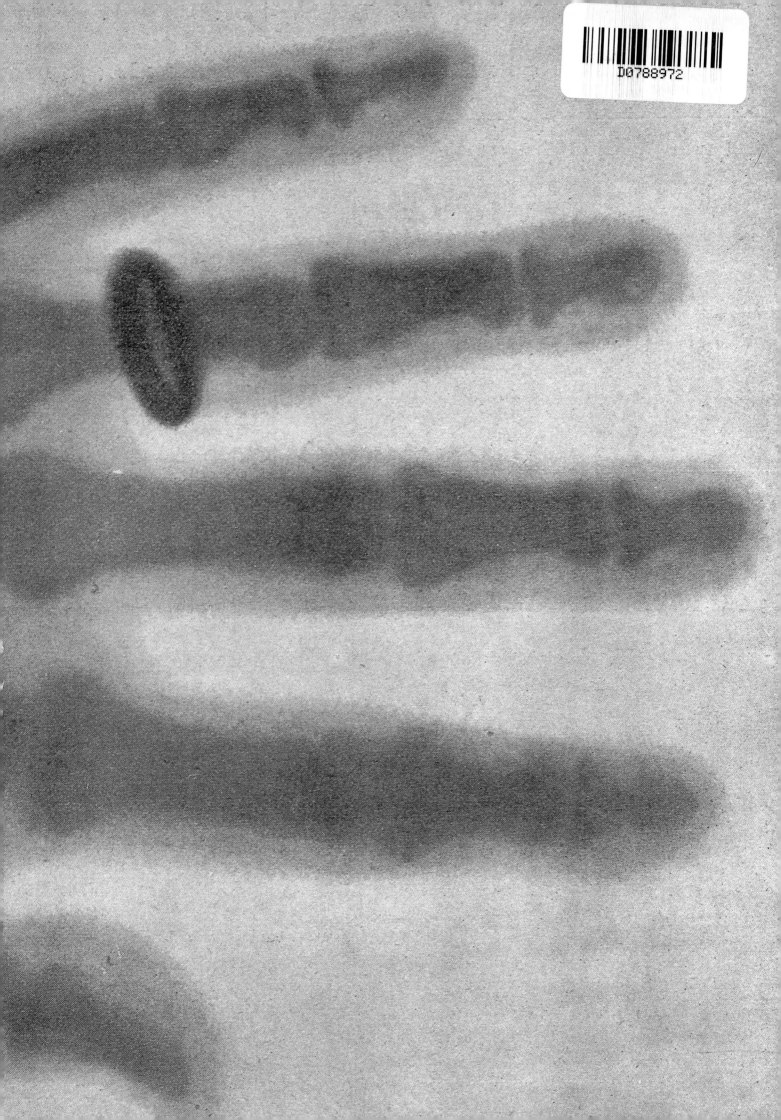

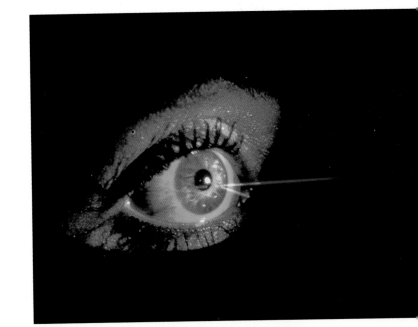

The History of Medicine

The History of

Medicine

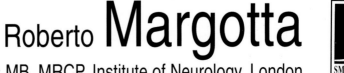

Roberto **Margotta**

Edited by Paul Lewis MB, MRCP, Institute of Neurology, London

SMITHMARK

CONTENTS

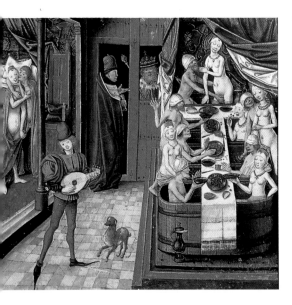

This edition published in 1996 by SMITHMARK Publishers, a division of U.S. Media Holdings Inc., 16 East 32nd Street, New York, NY 10016.

SMITHMARK books are available for bulk purchase for sales promotion and premium use. For details write or call the manager of special sales, SMITHMARK Publishers, 16 East 32nd Street, New York, NY 10016; (212) 532-6600

For copyright reasons this edition may not be sold outside the United States of America

Produced by Hamlyn, an imprint of Reed International Books Limited Michelin House, 81 Fulham Road, London SW3 6RB and Auckland, Melbourne, Singapore and Toronto

ISBN 0-7651-9905-X

Printed in Hong Kong

10 9 8 7 6 5 4 3 2 1

Based on an original text published in 1968 under the title *An Illustrated History of Medicine*, published by The Hamlyn Publishing Group, translated from the Italian *Medicina nei Secoli*, published in 1967 by Arnoldo Mondadori

The History of

Commissioning Editors Sian Facer and Jane McIntosh
Editor Anne Crane
Art Director Keith Martin
Design Manager Bryan Dunn
Art Editor Darren Kirk
Picture Researchers Jenny Faithfull, Claire Gouldstone, Julia Ruxton
Production Nick Thompson

5...

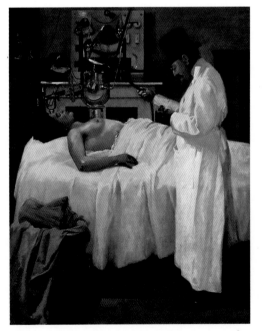

Medicine

FOREWORD

The purpose of this book is to present, in simple terms, a picture of the main stages of medicine in its evolution through the centuries. The story begins with the magic-imbued medicine of primitive man and concludes with modern achievements and thoughts on the future.

This book has two themes running through it. One is the continuous nature of medical development, which must be regarded as still at an early stage. Thus present-day theory and practice incorporates knowledge acquired over hundreds of years, while indeed many ancient ideas and some ancient forms of medicine survive to this day, especially in primitive societies. Despite the achievements of the last century, orthodox medical practice, unlike the scientific disciplines on which it is founded, remains by and large a matter of observation, opinion, and experience. A knowledge of the wrong turnings of the past is essential if the doctor of today is not to be arrogant in his overestimation of his powers. This applies not only to the clinician but also sometimes to the research worker, who, forgetting the heritage of William Harvey, starts from an incomplete set of findings and attempts to construct an edifice of knowledge based on Aristotelian logic and the power of argument, ignoring outside evidence and putting forward shaky new concepts – thereby committing a fundamental error and turning the clock back two thousand years.

The other theme is the importance of the act of faith on the part of the patient in his relationship with the doctor, something which is no less a vital element of healing today, when rational and radical cures are available for many diseases, than it was when medicine was entirely magical and empirical. Because this book deals only with the mainstream of medical development through the ages, such highly efficient and beneficial contemporary practices as osteopathy, whose rationale goes against the generally accepted concepts of anatomy, physiology and pathology, are not included.

Right: an inoculation session at a country clinic, 1868.

Pages 4 and 5: left, an illustration from a mediaeval manuscript, showing a communal bathing chamber; right, the first attempt to treat cancer with X-rays by Dr Chicotot, 1907. Painted by the doctor in 1908.

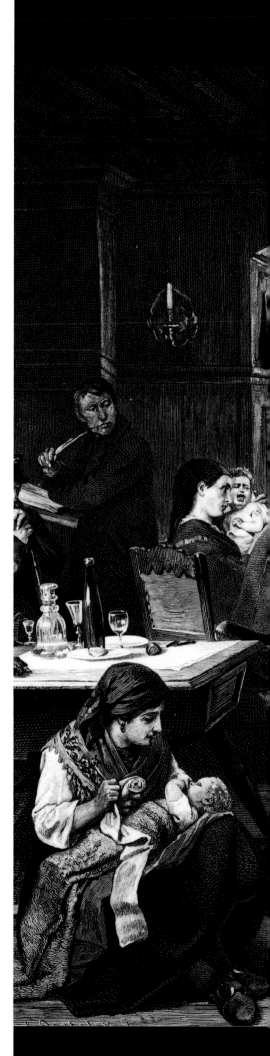

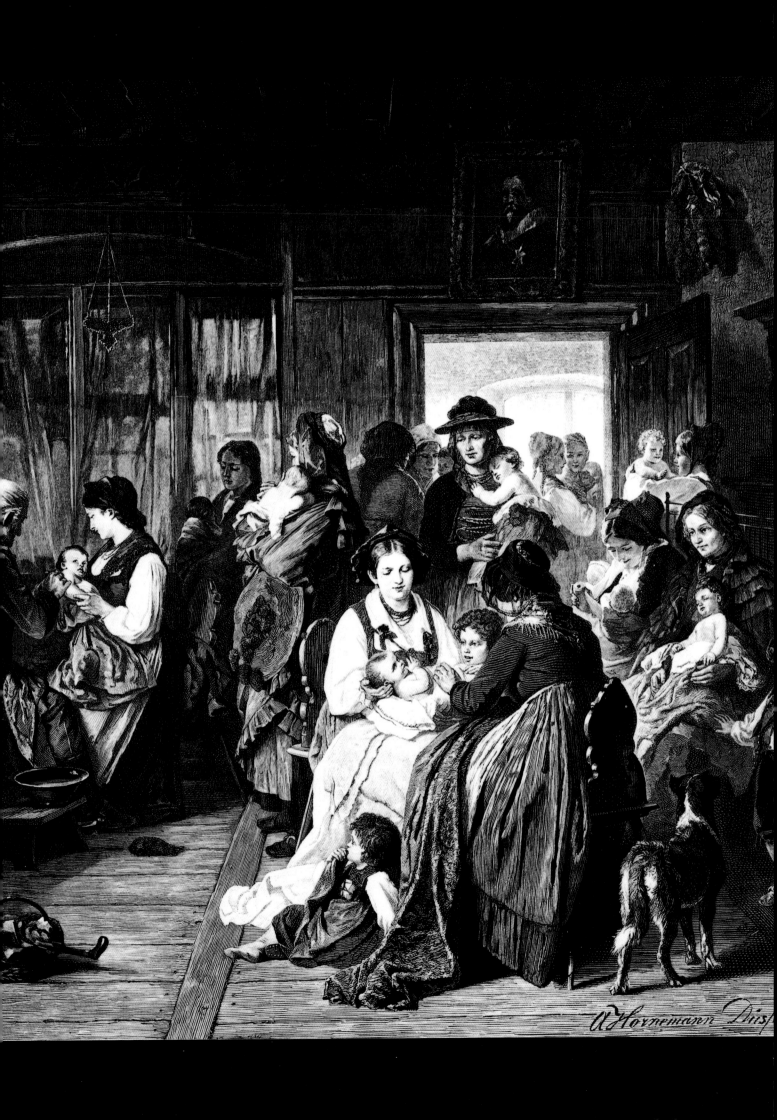

MAGIC AND EMPIRICAL MEDICINE

If medicine is the conscious attempt by man to fight disease, then it is as old as human consciousness itself. But what form the earliest medicine took must be entirely a matter for conjecture, in the absence of documentary evidence. However, in the light of nineteenth and twentieth century research, and the evidence of palaeontology and anthropology, it seems that it had its origins in magic and priestly practice.

Perhaps prehistoric man started by drawing a distinction between what could be seen and explained and what could not. Certainly fossil remains show evidence of such diseases as arthritis and tuberculosis as well as bone deformities caused by injury. On the one hand there were wounds from fighting other men and animals, and infestations with parasites, in all of which the cause was obvious and empirical treatment relatively easy; on the other hand there were diseases for which there was no apparent cause, which came from nowhere to threaten health and life. Thus in fear of disease and death man began to investigate the nature of life itself.

Powerless, he had to stand by and see his fellow-beings stricken by unknown forces. The conviction grew in him that the painful mysteries – like illness and death – were the work of demons, while there were undoubtedly kindly divinities too, responsible for the good and pleasant things in life. Other frightening and inexplicable things occurred besides pain and death, like storms and dark, moonless nights. Man associated these phenomena, too, with demons, supposing that they might be angry spirits of the dead or of animals killed in the hunt. It was as well, in any event to propitiate the supernatural powers by worship and sacrifice. Sorcerers came into being, who claimed to have knowledge of the stars, of the herbs of healing and poisons, and of the means to placate the evil demons, and so magic medicine evolved from practices which were instinctive and empirical.

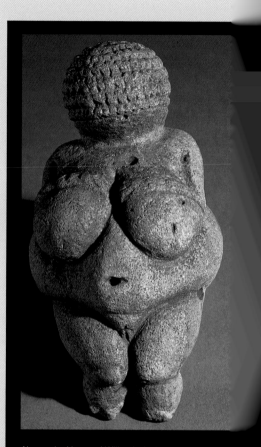

Above: the Venus of Willendorf, circa 20,000 BC, a sandstone statuette 10.5 cm (4 ¼ in) high, found in Austria and possibly the earliest known sculpture of the human figure. The Venus is considered to be a fertility figure.

It is likely that the functions of doctor and priest were then inseparable, as indeed they are today in primitive societies. In one cave in France, Les Trois Frères, a rock engraving has been found which dates back 17–20,000 years. It shows a doctor wearing a monstrous deer-mask over his face: he represents the archetypal sorcerer of a primitive community in any age. Animal masks were worn to frighten away the demon causing the illness and to impress the patient, so that he would have faith in the spells which were accompanied by suitably dramatic rituals, and in the medicines administered to him.

Sorcerers were magicians, weaving spells to make people sick and spells to make people well, and fashioning amulets to keep ill luck and illness at bay. As guardians of such vital secrets, they came to form a class apart. The rites they performed may seem charlatan, but their work had a certain relevance to modern medicine, for their lore was often gleaned from a study of nature, especially of the properties of plants and of animal poisons. The use, for example, of mandrake (which contains hyoscine) as a soporific and of antidotes to snake-bite goes back into the dim and distant past, anticipating two of the developments of medical science: sedatives and vaccination.

Above all, sorcerers were the first to practise trephining or perforation of the skull on living subjects. That patients survived the operation is known, since in many skulls, found in various parts of the world, the rims of the perforations are blunted, indicating clearly that healing processes later took place in the bone tissues. The sites of perforation suggest that surgery was practised for specific purposes, such as relieving headache or epilepsy. It is equally possible that the sorcerer wanted to remove something from the skull, which was plainly the home of important secrets. Perhaps it was a demon tormenting the subject; the operation was probably both ritual and therapeutic. Undoubtedly, some of the surgeons of prehistory had great technical ability. The oldest instruments were the sharpened edges of stones and flints, used to lance abscesses and let blood as well as for trephining.

The history of medicine has always been most closely connected with that of religion, for both after all work to the same end – the defence of the individual against evil forces – and, as religion took a more definite form in the earliest civilizations, so medicine gradually became established in the temples and sanctuaries of the gods.

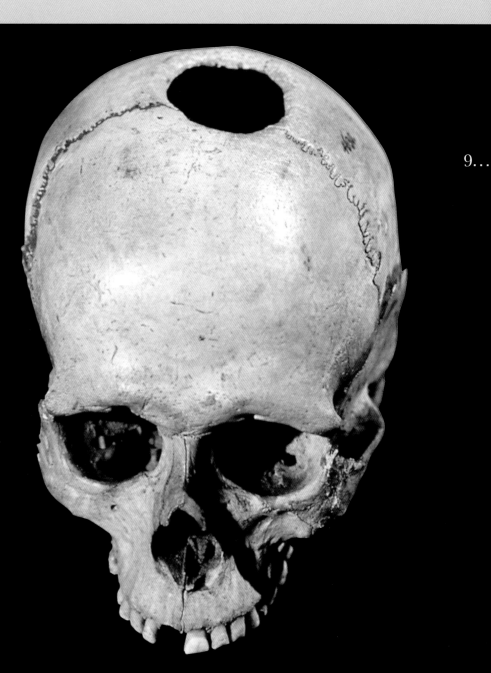

Medicine has its origins in magic and priestly practices. The dances of primitive peoples are often part of complex rites during which the supernatural is invoked.

9...

Right: a prehistoric trephined skull. Trephining holes may be round or square and vary in size from tiny holes to openings up to 5 cm (2 in) in diameter. Skulls have been found which show that the individual underwent the operation several times.

MESOPOTAMIA

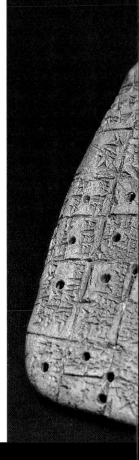

The Sumerians

The Sumerian civilisation, which flourished 6000 years ago at Ur in Mesopotamia, is the oldest one of whose medicine we have knowledge. It was based on the study of astrology, for the Sumerians believed that from birth man's destiny was ruled by the stars and they attempted to ascertain relationships between the movement of the stars and the seasons, and between changes of season and bodily disturbances.

Archaeologists have found clay tablets in Mesopotamia which were used by priests for writing out entire medical treatises. They thought that blood was the source of every vital function, with the liver as the collecting centre for the blood and so the seat of life; this is why the ancient heroes consulted the omens in the lobes of an animal liver, before embarking on great undertakings. This concept also gave rise to the idea that the continuation of life depended on the renewal of the blood by nourishment.

In 2000 BC, at the time of the great king Hammurabi, although the doctor-priests were answerable to the gods, surgeons were responsible to the civil authorities.

The Babylonian doctor

The Sumerian civilization was on the wane by 2000 BC, and was absorbed by that of the Assyrians and Babylonians who conquered Mesopotamia, which became the centre of Old World civilization, with a political system dominated by kings who claimed to be the intermediaries between the gods and the people. Astronomy and astrology, already important under the Sumerians, became even more important for it was essential to discover the will of the gods in order that the king might carry it out.

The king of the demon realm, the god of death and destruction was Nergal. When he visited mankind, he was heralded by Nasutar, the dreaded plague demon who in turn had a whole host of lesser demons at his beck and call, including *axaxuzu*, who produced jaundice, and *asukku*, who was the cause of consumption.

Many other illnesses were recognized, including different fevers, apoplexy and plague, and some clay tablets also give descriptions of diseases of the eyes, ears, skin and heart, rheumatism and of various venereal diseases. Toothache was thought to be caused by the gnawing of a worm, a common belief in Europe up till the eighteenth century. The demons were unleashed by the gods, in retribution for the sins of a man or a nation. When this happened, the doctor-priest stepped in and discovered the cause of the problem and then carried out the appropriate rites of exorcism and expiation.

Medicine among the Assyrians and Babylonians was the prerogative of the priests, who were answerable to the gods. But surgeons were laymen, answerable to the state for the operations they performed. The great king Hammurabi (1948–1905 BC) was the first in history to define the concept of the profession's civil and criminal liability; a copy of his Code is on a stele now in the Louvre in Paris. Some enactments laid down the scale of fees and the penalties for incompetence or negligence.

For example, Article 215 ordained: 'If the doctor performs a major operation or cures a diseased eye, he shall receive ten shekels of silver. If the patient is

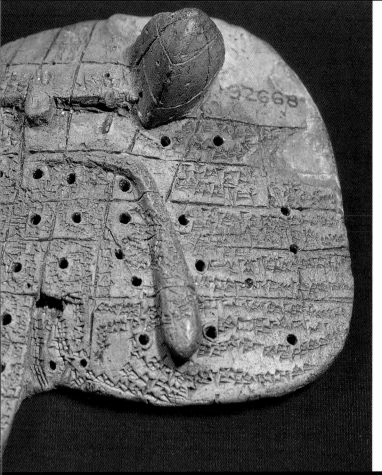

Left: a clay model of a sheep's liver, used for divination. First Babylonian dynasty, 1830–1530 BC.

a free man, he shall pay five shekels. If he is a slave, then his master shall pay two shekels on his behalf.' But if the patient lost his life or an eye in an operation, then the doctor's hands were cut off.

Although Assyrian and Babylonian doctors based their theories on magic symbolism, they were nevertheless acute observers of nature and so helped the advance of empirical medicine. For example, for eye trouble they prescribed a drink of beer and sliced onion. This is a perfectly valid, since an onion produces tears and tear fluid contains a bacterial substance, lysozyme. Then the eyes were massaged with olive oil. But finally a touch of ritual was added to deal with the evil spirit: a frog's bile mixed with sour milk was applied to the eyes. They prescribed a wide range of drugs for various complaints, including the fruits, flowers, leaves, roots and bark of such plants as the olive, laurel, asphodel, lotus and myrtle; and various organs from domestic and wild animals; and also a number of mineral substances such as iron, copper and aluminium. In addition, much use was made of the animal excreta, a practice common not only to primitive people, who perhaps adopted it to disgust and drive away the demon afflicting the sick patient, but also to European medicine until two hundred years ago.

Medicines were administered by Assyrian doctors in the form of pills, powders and enemas, and pessaries and suppositories were also used. On his rounds, the physician carried his case containing drugs, bandages and instruments, and after a consultation his findings would be recorded on clay tablets.

The descriptions of symptoms on the clay tablets are interesting. A typical one is for pulmonary tuberculosis: 'The patient coughs a lot, his saliva at times contains blood, his breathing sounds like a flute. His skin is clammy, but his feet are hot. He sweats profusely and his heart is in uproar. . . .'

Excavations in Babylon have also revealed large stone drains, probably part of a sewage system, and stone privies appear in the remains of this and other early Mediterranean civilizations. These primitive measures show a growing awareness of state responsibility for the health of its citizens.

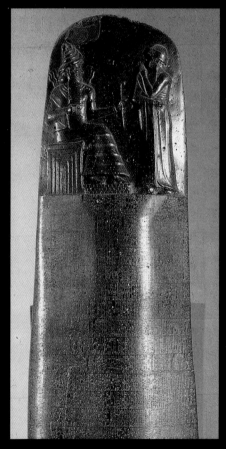

Above: the black stele inscribed with Hammurabi's professional code for surgeons, now in the Louvre, Paris. Although the punishments for negligence and incompetence laid down in the code are severe, there is evidence to show that they were not always strictly enforced.

THE MIDDLE EAST

In his *History*, Herodotus refers to the medicine of the peoples of the Nile valley. 'The art of medicine is thus divided: each physician applies himself to one disease only and not more. All places abound in physicians; some are for the eyes, others for the head, others for the teeth, others for the intestines, and others for internal disorders.' Diodorus Siculus, another Greek historian, records a practice which in a way anticipated modern welfare systems. 'In wartime and on journeys anywhere within Egypt, the sick are all treated free of charge, because doctors are paid by the state and scrupulous observance of the prescriptions drawn up by great doctors of the past is incumbent on them.'

As the centuries passed, medicine made little appreciable progress in the Nile valley. It was initiate medicine, practised for the purpose of ridding patients of demonic powers. All cures were revealed by the gods and codified by Thoth, known by the Greeks as Hermes Trismegistus, in secret books kept in the medical schools belonging to the temples of Sais at Heliopolis. They were books for initiates, that is to say priests. According to tradition, Thoth invented the sciences and the arts, knew the secrets of the gods and how to cause and cure illness. He is also said to have invented cursing by sympathetic magic.

Knowledge of Egyptian medicine comes mainly from what are called the medical papyri, writings exclusively medical in content. The papyri found by Georg Ebers and Edwin Smith are the most interesting. That of Ebers, discovered at Luxor in 1873, which can be dated to the period 1553–1550 BC, is a collection of texts which probably originated in the old empire (3300–2360 BC), from the time of the first eight dynasties whose rulers built the pyramids of Cheops, Chefren and Mycerinus.

Above: an Egyptian statue inscribed with magical texts for healing, from the Thirtieth Dynasty or early Ptolemaic period, c.380–300 BC.

Until the discovery of the medical papyri in the late nineteenth century, especially those found by Georg Ebers and Edwin Smith, knowledge of Egyptian medicine came mainly from the writings of the Greeks and Romans, among them Homer, Herodotus, Hippocrates and Pliny. The Egyptian doctors a used a huge variety of drugs, including opium and hemlock.

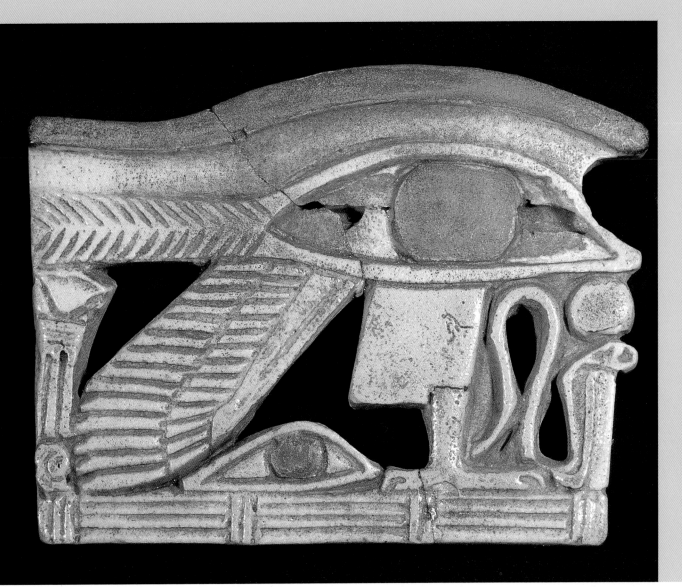

Imhotep lived during the third dynasty. He was famous as an architect and as a pyramid builder, but he was also a great doctor; he was deified by the Egyptians, and the Greeks identified him with Asklepios, now more commonly known by his Latin name Aesculapius, their god of medicine. It may well be that some of the prescriptions in the Ebers papyrus were originated by Imhotep.

The earlier papyrus found by Smith gives instructions for the treatment of wounds, fractures and dislocations. For fractures the Egyptians used birch splints with bandages bound over them, and a method for treating a dislocated jaw was not unlike that used today. Lesions on the right or left sides of the head were observed to be associated with paralysis on the opposite side of the body. Prognostic statements were also recorded: 'I will cure this disease' was usually recorded if the outcome appeared favourable; 'Nothing can be done in this case', if doubtful, or 'The patient will die', if hopeless.

Unlike the Assyrians and Babylonians, who thought of the liver as the seat of life, the Egyptians regarded respiration as the most important vital function. They knew that the heart was the centre of the circulation, but supposed that the circulation depended on breathing. They recognized various complaints affecting the heart, abdomen and eyes, and also angina pectoris, disorders of the bladder and various kinds of swelling.

Above: the Eye of Horus, an amulet made of enamel and glazed pottery dating from the Late Dynastic period, c.600 BC.

One of the many treatments in the Ebers papyrus runs: 'In the case of a tumour affecting a vessel in the form of a callosity which is stone-like to the touch, I would say it is a tumour of the vessels suitable for treatment by surgery. After surgery, cauterize the wound, lest it bleed too much.' When physicians went visiting, they took their patients' pulses, examined their bodies and went through a process of auscultation by laying an ear to the shoulder blades and chest.

Considering the mummies and the refined embalming techniques used in the Nile valley, it might be thought that Egyptian medical men were strong on anatomy. In fact they were, but only to a certain level; anatomy seems to have been learned from a study of animals, judging by hieroglyphs, that for 'heart' being shaped like that of a cow, 'throat' like the head and windpipe of cattle, and 'uterus' being bicornuate, unlike that of the human female. But embalming was not done by the priest-doctors but by those who worked in the house of death, who formed another distinct class.

Herodotus describes the technique of embalming: the brain was removed by a hook inserted through the nose, and the brain cavity cleaned with the utmost care. The body was opened by means of long vertical incision, and when the internal organs had been removed it was washed several times over with infusions of aromatic herbs and then filled with spices of all kinds. The opening was then sewn up and the body was immersed for a certain time in a special solution. After this, it was washed again and swathed in linen bands impregnated with bituminous substances, which ensured it would remain in a perfect state of preservation. In fact, preservation is often so good that under a microscope tissue sections shows fine detail and sometimes evidence of disease.

right. Anubis, the Egyptian god of the dead and the patron god of embalmers, embalming a body. A wall painting from the tomb of Sennedjem, New Kingdom, Nineteenth Dynasty, circa 1320–1200 BC.

Rules for diet, body cleanliness and child welfare were set out in the book of Leviticus.

The health laws of the Israelites

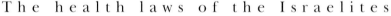

For the ancient Hebrews, disease was not due to a demon or evil spirit or to spells cast by jealous fellow men, but represented God's wrath at the sins of men. Health could never fail as long as the Ten Commandments were observed. In order to get well, a sick man had to ask the priests to intercede on his behalf, since they were the arbiters of the law of Moses and did more health work than the doctors.

By attesting belief in one God, the giver of good health and bad, Mosaic law had the power to overcome superstition and magic practices, though these did persist to a certain extent. It was faith and faith alone that brought health to the body and salvation to the soul. Since to be unclean was the worst sin of all, the rules of hygiene laid down in the scriptures aimed to make men clean in the eyes of God. Physical and moral purity were thus equated.

In the book of Leviticus there is an exemplary code of health (V, 2-3): 'A man may have touched what has been killed by a wild beast or has fallen dead . . . or some other unclean thing, unaware of his defilement at the time: yet he has incurred guilt by the fault. Or he has touched some defilement of the human body; there are many such; he may be unaware of it till afterwards, but he has incurred guilt . . .' A purifying bath would cleanse him of this guilt before he could enter the Temple.

During menstruation, a woman was unclean and could not carry out religious duties in the temple, or have intercourse with her husband. When the menstrual flow ceased she had to be purified by a ritual bath, and before being immersed naked in the water, her body had to be carefully washed. Every community, no matter how small, always built a ritual bath as well as a synagogue. The list of people who were unclean included those with infectious diseases

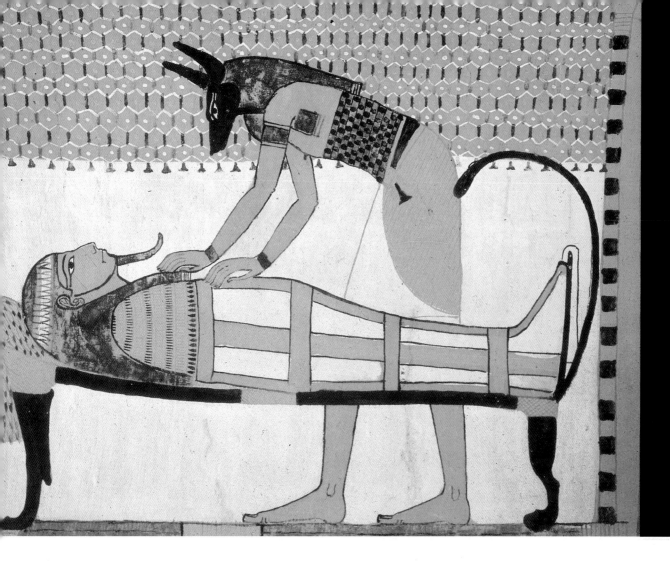

such as gonorrhoea and leprosy, who made anything or any individual they touched unclean as well. It was also a religious duty to wash the hands before meals; washing them after meals was regarded as a sign of respect to others rather than as a religious one. Regulations for the control of contagious disease represented the first compulsory health enactments. When an epidemic was raging, alarms were sounded and people who caught the disease were isolated and their clothing and houses disinfected.

The ancient Jewish surgeons had great skill. They performed operations for anal fistula, for imperforate anus in the newborn, Caesarean section, and treated dislocations and fractures by rational methods. The practice of circumcision was so much a part of ancient tradition that it was performed with stone tools even after metal ones had come into common use. Our knowledge of Jewish surgery comes from the Talmud, which also contains accurate descriptions of many diseases, including jaundice and diphtheria.

Persian medicine

In the Persian sacred book, the *Avesta,* medicine was a weapon in the fight against demons.

Ancient Persian medicine may have shared a common origin with Jewish medicine, for it too placed emphasis on personal and communal hygiene. Health depended on the god of light and good, Ahura Mazda, and medicine was entirely in the hands of his followers. A professional code is laid down in the *Vendidad,* stipulating training requirements, fees and penalties for malpractice. Surgeons as well as physicians existed at this period, for in the writings of Firdausi, who lived around AD 1000, are to be found descriptions of doctors in ancient Persia who healed with the knife, as well as accounts of successful Caesarean section. Herodotus recorded other practices, such as segregating the sick and those suffering from contagious disease.

ANCIENT INDIAN MEDICINE

The first period of Indian medicine began with the Hindu invasion of the Punjab in about 1500 BC. It was during this period that the books of *Veda* (learning) were composed. They included the *Ayurveda* (Veda of long life), which was concerned particularly with medicine. As these are sacred texts revealed by divine beings, the history in them is interwoven with legend.

The Vedic period was followed around the beginning of the ninth century BC by the Brahminical period, which marked a peak in Indian medicine. The two great Hindu doctors, Charaka and Susruta, whose writings formed the groundwork for all subsequent systems of Indian medicine, belong to this period. The *Charaka Samhita*, which is arranged in eight books, is set out in the form of a dialogue between master and pupil, and is to medicine what the *Susruta Samhita*, which is less accurate but shows fair knowledge of human anatomy, is to surgery.

The main feature of medical thinking in ancient India was a tendency to construct a highly compartmentalised system, with a niche for every concept. Their medical works are of composite nature, like encyclopedias. For this reason scholars have been unable to date their range of concepts and precepts, or to pick out essentially Indian ideas from those derived from other civilizations.

Ancient Hindu medicine was strong in surgery and weak in anatomy, a subject which might be expected to be fundamental to surgery. This was probably due to the religious laws which forbade the use of a knife on a dead body. In order to study the internal organs, Susruta advised doctors to immerse a body in a basket in the river; after seven days of decomposition, the organs could be viewed simply by poking away the overlying skin and other soft tissues.

Right: a giant having a tooth pulled out. A Buddhist bas-relief from Bharut, dating from the second century BC.

Apart from this, ancient Indian texts are devoid of anatomical references.

A field in which the ancient Indians were centuries ahead was plastic surgery. Rhinoplasty, for reshaping the nose, was very widely practised. It was not so much a question of aesthetics, to improve on nature, as a rebuilding operation since adultery was punishable in India by cutting off the nose and the operation was devised as an attempt to restore the normal appearance of those who suffered this penalty.

Susruta explains how the surgeon worked. From the leaf of a plant he cut a piece the size of the missing nose. This he laid on the patient's cheek and cutting round it removed a piece of skin of the same size. Then the surgeon applied this piece to the nose stump, from which the skin had been removed, and sewed it on. After that, he put two pieces of hollow reed into the nostrils so that the patient could breathe easily. If the nose was now too big, he cut it off and started again.

Many other surgical procedures are described in Susruta's book, including operations on anal fistulas and neck tumours, and tonsillectomy, lithotomy, lancing of abscesses and amputation of limbs. A detailed list of 121 surgical instruments is given, including knives, scalpels, bistouries, saws, scissors, forceps for extracting teeth and others for extracting foreign bodies from nose and ear, three different kinds of needle for suturing, catheters and syringes. A section is devoted to the treatment of fractures with bamboo splints.

Diagnostic technique was also of a relatively high standard. Doctors inspected and palpated the patient, listened to his heart, lungs and abdomen,

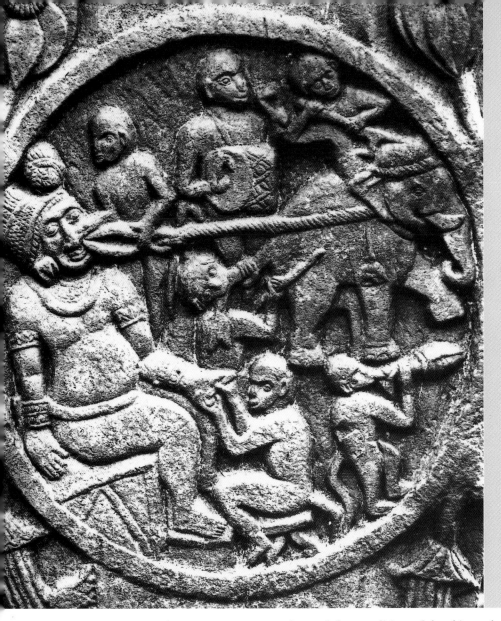

The ancient Indians were centuries ahead of all other civilisations in the field of plastic surgery, performing operations to restore the nose.

and noted the condition of the skin and tongue. Many illnesses were attributed to imbalance between the three physical humours – spirit, bile and phlegm. Besides these there were moral humours, disturbance of which could also underlie physical illness, an idea echoed in the present-day concept of psychosomatic disease. Ancient medical treatises give very accurate descriptions of the symptoms of diabetes and tuberculosis and of contagious diseases, especially smallpox. The Indians of that time knew that malaria was a consequence of mosquito bites, and in a Sanskrit text, predating Susruta, the role of plague carrier was ascribed to rats. Apart from a number of magical practices, Indian therapy was based on purgatives, enemas, emetics, blood-letting by leeches, steam baths, inhalations and sternutatories (preparations to cause sneezing – which was believed to clear the head). Susruta lists 760 medicinal plants, including *Atropa belladonna* (deadly nightshade) and *Cannabis indica* (Indian hemp) to induce stupor, and *Rauwolfia serpentina* for sedation.

An extremely important part is played in Indian medicine by the strict hygiene rules of the Brahmin religion. A largely vegetarian diet is recommended and abstention from alcohol is ordained, and there is great emphasis on cleanliness, with much bathing and the immediate removal of excreta and other waste from the house.

The third period of Hindu medicine dates from AD 664, after the Moslem conquest of India, and resulted in the introduction of Arab medicine to India. At the same time, Ayurvedic medicine persisted and in fact survives to the present day, being practised in innumerable villages by doctors called *kaviraj.*

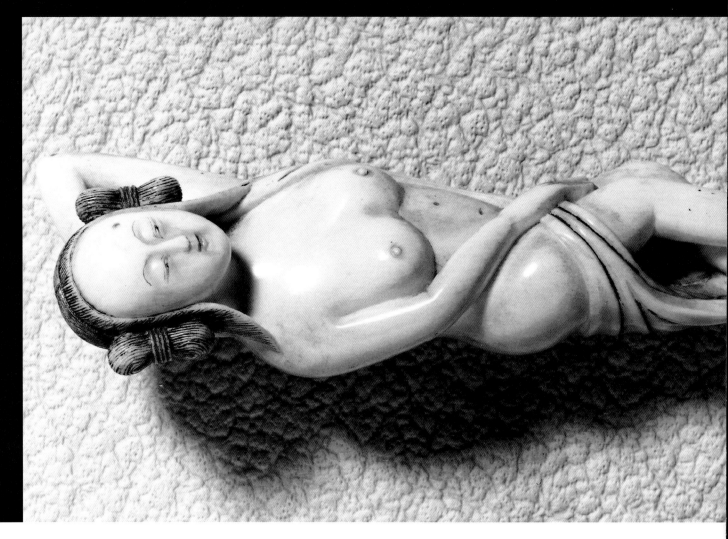

TRADITIONAL CHINESE MEDICINE

Above: an ivory diagnostic statuette. It was considered bad form for a male doctor to examine a female patient intimately, so women would take a statuette to their doctor and use it to indicate the site of the problem.

While the Egyptian pharaohs were building pyramids, the ancient Chinese emperors were obsessed with medicine. Yet the history of China bears some resemblance to that of Egypt, in that it embraced a series of dynasties dating back to Shen Nung, a legendary emperor who is said to have ruled from 2838–2698 BC. This enlightened ruler was looked upon as the inventor of medicine, under the inspiration of Pan Ku, the god to whom the creation of the world was attributed in Taoist legend: chaos was overcome and order established on the basis of two opposite poles, *yin* and *yang*.

The *yang* principle was positive, active and masculine, as signified by the sky, light, might, hardness, warmth and dryness, and also the left side. The *yin* principle on the other hand was negative, being passive and feminine, as signified by the moon, earth, darkness, weakness, cold and moisture and the right side. Chinese medicine was based on these two principles; *yin* and *yang* together with the blood constituted the vital substance that circulated in the body. Illness was held to be caused by imbalance of the two principles, while death supervened when they ceased to flow.

A particular contribution of Shen Nung to Chinese medicine was his *Pen T'sao Ching* or Herbal. This little book lists 365 herbs, prescriptions and poisons in three volumes. Quite a few of the prescriptions found in this herbal and its

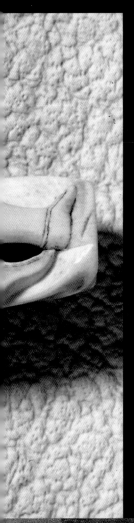

successors are common to modern therapy, for example, opium as a narcotic, rhubarb as a laxative, flowers of artemisia for worms, rauwolfia for sedation, kaolin for diarrhoea, ephedrine for asthma and chaulmoogra oil for leprosy. Following it a succession of similar works appeared, culminating in the *Pen T'sao Kang Mu* or Great Herbal (AD 1552) of Li Shi-Chen, which describes 1,871 drugs in fifty-two volumes and took twenty-seven years to compile.

In addition to the prescriptions derived from Shen Nung, the ancient Chinese made use of other treatments which are still found in modern pharmacopoeias, such as sodium sulphate for purging and iron for anaemia, as well as essentially Chinese preparations such as ones containing ginseng. They also took the first steps to immunize against smallpox, introducing pustular crusts in powder form into the nostrils (the left nostril for boys, the right for girls).

Another emperor with an important place in medicine was Hwang Ti (2698–2598 BC), to whom is ascribed the *Nei Ching* or Book of Medicine, the most ancient as well as the greatest Chinese medical work, and one that is still studied in China. It was transmitted orally for centuries, and is thought to have been first written down in the third century BC. One passage from it states: 'All the blood of the human body is under the control of the heart and regulated by it. The blood current flows continuously in a circle and never stops; it cannot but flow ceaselessly like the current of a river or the sun and the moon in their courses.' These are superficially remarkable statements, considering that ancient Chinese understanding of anatomy was limited. Dissection of the dead, while generally prohibited (for a man had to die with his body whole if he was to join his ancestors), seems to have been attempted, judging by some anatomical measurements given in the book. The suggestion has been made that it was the prerogative of the Chinese emperors as absolute rulers to conduct anatomical investigations. More probably, Hwang Ti's statement about the circulation of the blood should be regarded as a remarkable guess.

Chinese doctors did not delve into the medical histories of their patients, or go in for full physical examinations. In diagnosis, they concentrated on examining the pulse, taking it in many ways and producing a long list of variations, each with its own prognostic significance. For the pulse indicated the flow of the vital element, formed from the union of *yin* and *yang* with the blood.

The most famous Chinese surgeon was Hua T'o, who lived about the second century AD. Before performing an operation, incision or amputation, Hua T'o is said to have made the patient insensible of pain by administering a narcotic brew he had made himself. Some eight centuries before Hua T'o, the practice of castration was widespread in China and many doctors specialized in it, to provide eunuchs for the emperors' service. Then, too, surgeons used to dull pain before the operation by using anaesthetic substances; none of the old texts give details of the ingredients, but in more recent times a hot decoction of pepper pods was used, applied to the genitals. For the operation itself, the penis and scrotum were tied together with a strip of silk, and a semi-circular knife was used to sever them in front of the pubis. To stop the bleeding, a styptic powder of rock alum and resin was applied. The surgeon next put a plug of wood in the urethra. If the patient survived, he was ready three months later for his duties as guardian of the imperial concubines.

Another practice which persisted into this century was the binding of the feet of upper-class women. The victims of this custom, imposed from a misguided sense of aesthetics, were not given the option of refusal. While they were still too young to resist, they had to undergo tight and painful bandaging, to turn the toes down and hold up the instep, with permanent deformity.

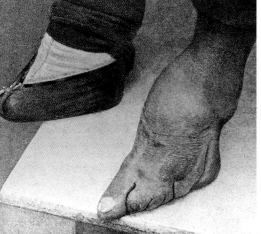

Above: the feet of an upper-class woman, permanently misshapen and disabled by foot binding. For centuries, tiny feet were regarded by the Chinese as a woman's most attractive feature.

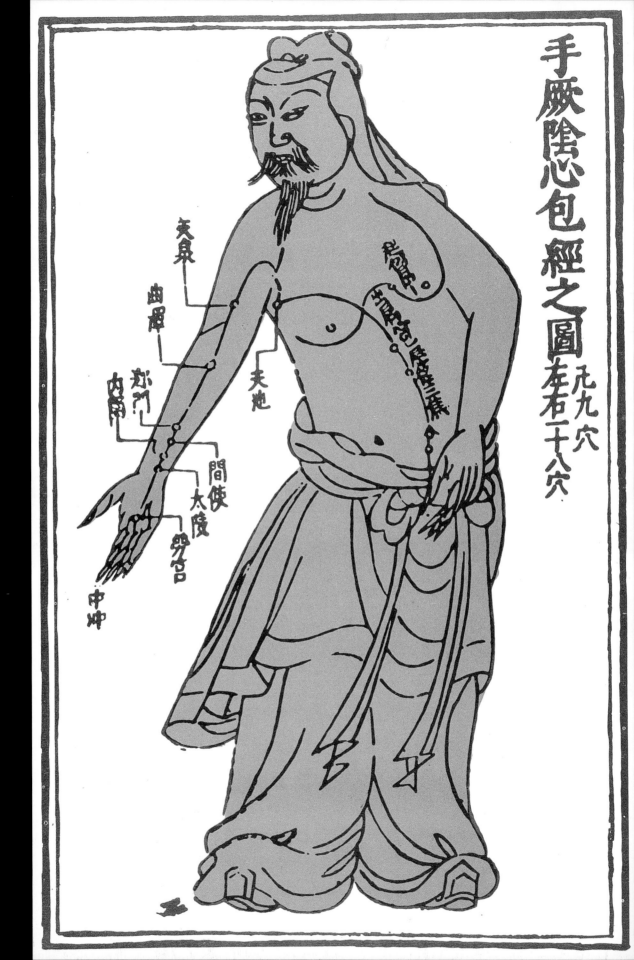

手厥陰心包經之圖左右二十八穴凡九穴

天泉

曲澤

郄門

內關

間使

太陵

勞宮

中沖

天池

20

The most typically Chinese medical practice was acupuncture. It consists in pricking the patient's skin with needles of gold, silver or iron, cold or hot, of various lengths from 2.5–28 cm (1–10 in). The idea was to remove any obstruction in the *chin*, *loh* or *sun*, the vessels carrying the two vital principles, blood and air. Old treatises name some 365 points for acupuncture. Specialists taught their pupils by means of metal statuettes, pricked all over with holes at the points of puncture.

In the following centuries, Chinese medicine came to a standstill because of people's veneration for the wisdom of their ancestors. It was not until the thirteenth century that another major advance took place. In 1247, the judge Sung Tz'u compiled the *Hsi Yüan Lu*, the standard treatise on law and medicine. It was intended for the magistrates and contained information on ascertaining the cause of death from a careful study of the deceased: accurate descriptions were given of signs to distinguish death by drowning, poisoning, strangling, stabbing and bludgeoning. As well as establishing diagnostic methods to distinguish murder from suicide, the work gave instructions on artificial respiration and antidotes to poisons.

Then, while science and learning advanced in Europe, Chinese medicine remained at a standstill. The teachings inherited from the ancients were so scrupulously revered that all progress was impeded. European medicine did not reach China until the nineteenth century.

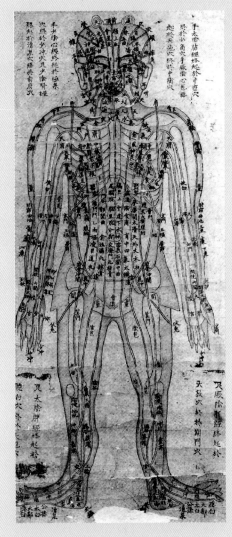

Right: *Fu-jen Ming-t'ang t'u* acupuncture chart. Acupuncture charts date from the T'ang Dynasty (AD 618–906) or possibly even earlier.

21...

Left: an acupuncture chart, dating from the Ming Dynasty (AD 1368–1644), and showing the puncture points and describing their significance.

The greatest achievements of ancient Chinese medicine were a series of herbals culminating in the *Pen T'sao Kang Mu* or Great Herbal of AD 1552, which ran to fifty-two volumes.

Japan

About the fourth century AD, Chinese civilization penetrated Japan, and for many centuries it entirely dominated the islands, its medicine supplanting native practices. The first attempts to reduce Chinese influence came in the sixteenth century, the greatest reformer being the physician Tokuhon Nagata (1512–1630), while the arrival of the Portuguese in 1542 introduced European medicine, which the Japanese adopted as avidly as they had adopted Chinese methods before.

Little is known of Japanese medicine in the days before the Chinese arrived, although old legends indicate rudimentary anatomical knowledge and a theory of disease based on evil spirits and divine influences.

ANCIENT GREECE

Surgeons at the siege of Troy

Ancient Aegean civilization began around 3000 BC with the conquest of the Greek islands by the races inhabiting the eastern shores of the Mediterranean. Various Oriental influences were fused into pre-Hellenic culture and at the same time transmuted by the process of separation from Asia.

Hellenic medicine developed with philosophy, disciplined by strict criticism, and healing for the first time became a science as well as an art, practised not by a priestly caste but by laymen who replaced magic by enquiry. The most ancient source of information about the medicine of the Greeks is the work of Homer. A doctor was a respected figure; Homer wrote: 'He is worth many lives, being unequalled in removing arrows from wounds and healing them with herb ointments'.

In the *Iliad*, Homer refers to the removal of arrowheads and javelins, and to bandaging, compresses, methods of stopping bleeding and of curing wounds with balm, and to medicines made of herbal extracts. Wine and other liquids are also used to revive the injured. Without a doubt the medical information Homer gives must reflect contemporary practice in the pre–Hellenic civilisations of Crete and the Aegean.

Like most early peoples, the Greeks recognized the importance of blood though not its true functions. The practice of bleeding was used then and for centuries later for various complaints, either by cutting veins or by cupping.

Above: a detail from a Greek vase showing a doctor treating a patient.

Hellenic medicine developed with philosophy, and healing for the first time became a science as well as an art.

The temples of Aesculapius

Despite the frequent references in the *Iliad* to the gods and the prayers of the dying, it is clear that medicine at the time of Homer was not based on magic, but was an independent discipline practised by experts who earned a living from it. But as time went by Oriental influences on Greek culture became increasingly marked; in consequence medicine became more and more priestly and literature after Homer contains an increasing number of incantations and references to demons, soothsayers and omens.

Many of the Greek gods came to be identified with healing. Not only Apollo, Artemis, Athene and Aphrodite but also the gods of the underworld were able to cure or avert disease. The cult of Aesculapius may well have developed from the worship of one of these deities, for his symbol, the serpent, is a very ancient representation of underworld forces and was a sacred sign of the god of healing among the Semitic tribes of Asia Minor. It is not known if Aesculapius really lived and was a doctor deified after death. It is said that while on earth, he was the father of a large family, including Panacea, who had a cure for everything, and Hygiea whose domain was public health.

It was probably around 770 BC that the first Aesculapian sanctuaries, dedicated to the god of medicine, were built, and the serpent cult began to spread, although the serpent was already very important in magic medicine. The temple-building movement developed rapidly; over three hundred sites have been mentioned by classical authors. These temples were usually well situated with woods and springs of water, perhaps with mineral properties, and commanding splendid views, the most famous being at Epidaurus, Cnidus, Cos, Athens, Pergamon and Cyrene. People were still visiting them in the fifth century AD. Among the Greeks, unlike other ancient peoples, religion was a poetic

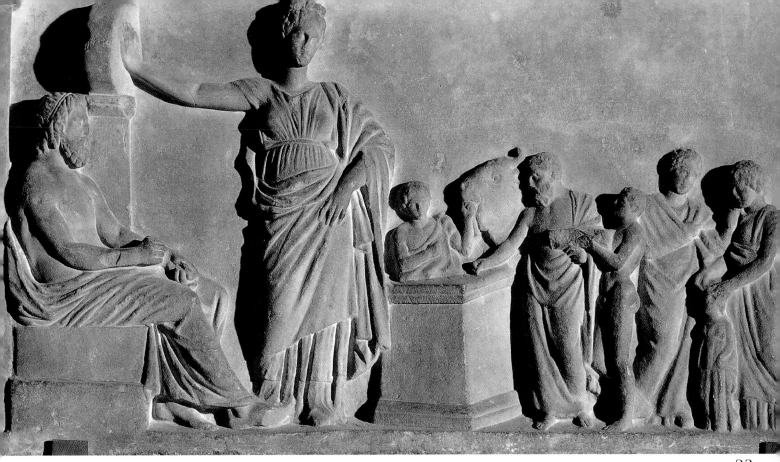

Above: Aesculapius with his children. His sons were the gods of surgeons and physicans while his daughters were goddesses of healing and health.

Below: Aesculapius with his staff round which twists the serpent, the ancient symbol of medicine.

myth, never infringing freedom to criticize and explore nature, and the priests were never a special caste. They worked for gain. When the treatment by lay doctors failed, people turned to Aesculapian sanctuaries for help.

Treatment at the sanctuaries was conservative and was based on bathing and fasting. Once patients had been purified and were ready to approach the altar, a propitiation ceremony was held and the sick were admitted to the inner-most precinct, the *abaton*. There, wrapped in blankets, they lay down on sheepskins and slumbered, exhausted from fasting and drugged with sleeping draughts. Then came the main part of the treatment: as soon as the patients were asleep, the priests started passing in and out among the beds, followed by the sacred serpents, which licked the sores of the sleeping patients. On waking, each patient had to give an account of what he had dreamed. A priest then explained the meaning of it to him and prescribed the appropriate treatment. A cure resulted sometimes, but the priests had a ready reply if there was no improvement; the patient had not done exactly as he had been told to, or had simply lacked faith in their treatment.

Before he left the sanctuary the sick man would offer money and a votive tablet with his name, affliction and treatment recorded on it. The tablets were hung on the walls of the temple and no doubt imbued trust in newcomers to the sanctuary. Today they are of interest for their recognizable depiction of various diseases, including breast cancer, and for their accounts of cures.

However, in spite of the criticism and the growing influence of lay medicine, priestly medicine spread throughout Greece in the fifth century BC and in fact was in common practice up to the fourth or fifth centuries AD, when the cult of Aesculapius is sometimes found mingled with that of Christian saints.

Lay medicine

It was the cult of Aesculapius that made the Greeks begin to lay particular stress on one aspect of illness – the hope and anxiety of patients about their recovery. It could be said that psychotherapy, freed from exorcism, was initiated in the sanctuaries. As time went by, the priests moved further and further from purely ritual treatment. Lay medicine was practised from the earliest times alongside this temple system. From the sixth century BC, medicine had professional status. Newly trained students applied for a licence to practise from a council which was only granted when the standing of the student's school had been taken into account. Practitioners could open a surgery in which they could receive and treat patients and charge fees.

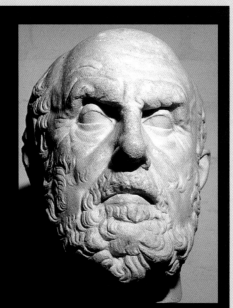

...24

Above: Pythagoras, the most important founder of the medical school at Croton, where the first truly scientific studies on anatomy and physiology were carried out.

The Graeco-Italic school – the dawn of scientific medicine

The Greeks had enquiring minds, and made a fresh approach to the problems life presented. Man and nature were the subjects of their scrutiny; thus the first philosophers were pre-eminently biologists and naturalists. By philosophy, the Greeks meant the attempt to understand man and the world; their aim was to devise a good way of life and then to let everyone live it.

The Graeco-Italic school was a great philosophic school, founded by Pythagoras (580–489 BC), which provided the most important basis of scientific medicine. It is associated with the town of Croton in southern Italy, which already had a flourishing medical school before Pythagoras arrived from Greece. Here, Pythagoras carried out much research, infusing new life into the school and ensuring its survival by instituting an association of very strict rules for initiates. Rather in the style of a secret society, adepts swore loyalty to the leader and promised not to betray any of their esoteric knowledge to the uninitiated. Before Pythagoras the concept of disease was shrouded by a supernatural veil. With his teaching, it was seen by the light of the rising star of science. The principle of harmony and proportion governing the universe, the macrocosm, was reflected in the microcosm of the human organism.

The most famous doctor of the Croton school was Alcmaeon, a younger contemporary of Pythagoras, who gave medicine the true dignity of a science. He discovered the optic nerves and the Eustachian tube of the ear, and was the first to assert that the brain was the seat of the intellect and the senses. He recognized three main factors affecting the sight: external light, internal fire and liquid contained in the eye. This master of anatomy and physiology also made some observations on the circulation and distinguished veins from arteries. He investigated the function disturbances caused by brain injuries and proposed a long-accepted explanation of sleep and death. Camillo Golgi, the Italian Nobel prizewinner noted, as late as 1910, that Alcmaeon's theory was 'generally held to this very day, in the form of cerebral anaemia'. Alcmaeon in fact maintained that sleep occurred when the blood ebbed from the brain into the veins, and that when this outflow was complete and one-way only, death ensued.

The book *On nature* contained the sum of Alcmaeon's learning. It is important because it offered the Greeks a plausible explanation for the nature of disease and suggested means of prevention and cure, without recourse to the supernatural. According to Alcmaeon, health and ill-health depended on pairs of elemental opposites, like hot and cold, wet and dry, sweet and sour, and so on; disease was due to some disturbance in their balance. The desire to conquer disease was first embodied in concrete form when he listed the potential sources of disharmony: the nature of the individual, malnutrition, irregular or inadequate diet, and external factors such as climate and altitude. Today this may seem rather slight, but people then may have thought that it needed only a few more discoveries for the battle against disease to be won.

A notable contribution was made by another of the Graeco-Italic school, Empedocles of Agrigentum (c.500–430 BC), who held an Olympian view of the laws governing the universe. He thought that the world was made of four elements, which were formed and unalterable and which he called the root of all things – earth, air, fire and water. His teaching led to the heart being regarded as the centre of the circulatory system: blood flowing continuously to and from the heart while the pneuma, or breath of life, was distributed throughout the body by the blood vessels. He believed that breathing was not confined to the lungs, but also took place through the pores of the skin.

It can be said that the practicality of the Greeks in this and other medical matters was one of the results of the influence of pre-Socratic philosophy and in particular of the teachings of the school of Pythagoras. These placed especial emphasis on the direct observation of nature and inductive reasoning and on investigation into the cause and meaning of life. The Pythagorean school also elaborated the doctrine of the four elements and corresponding humours, which was to dominate pathology for centuries.

While the Graeco-Italic school developed in southern Italy and Sicily, other important medical schools flourished at Cyrene in North Africa, at Cnidus at the southern tip of Asia Minor, and on the islands of Rhodes and Cos. The school at Cos was to become the most famous. Here teaching was based closely on diagnosis and examination and doctors concerned themselves not so much with discussion of the causes of disease as with the prognosis of the individual patient. Important too was the recognition for the first time of diseases as general conditions not limited to a particular organ or part of the body while emphasis on diseases with a periodic nature led to the doctrine of crisis and critical days – reflecting the old Babylonian astrological concepts. Thus various factors, including traditional empirical medicine, Assyro-Babylonian astronomy and Jewish and Egyptian sanitary laws, combined to form the foundations of the work of the greatest teacher of Cos – Hippocrates.

Empedocles of Agrigentum believed that the world was made of four elements which were formed and unalterable and which he described as the root of all things – earth, air, fire and water.

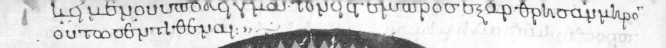

ὁμωολὴ μηροῦ. ἡ δ γ᾽ ἀντηοορ γαρι
ιλιαωαγι λοο᾽ ἡ τω ρ᾽μρ̣ ιολιω ρ̣τ δ̣ιαγ
τοῦ-ϑϑ μαρόφου ἰατρου γ᾽ ρ ο μωρ̣ ἡ
ἡω ἡ γ᾽ὁ ϑμωρ̣ω᾽ μϑ̣ρ̣ω ̣ολ ι ω ϑ ̣ ̣

Above: treatment for a leg using the Hippocratic bench. From an eleventh-century codex: *Commentaries of Apollonius of Chition on the Peri arthron of Hippocrates.*

'I swear by Apollo the healer, by Aesculapius, by health and all the powers of healing . . . that I will use my power to help the sick to the best of my ability and judgment.' From the Hippocratic Oath.

HIPPOCRATES, FATHER OF MEDICINE

A great plane tree still stands on the island of Cos, in the Aegean, under which, it is said, young men were formally initiated into the art of medicine as long ago as the end of the fifth century BC. With their fellows and elders clustered around, they would take an oath which is now known as the Hippocratic Oath, renowned through the centuries for setting a high standard of professional conduct. In the fifth century BC it symbolized the spirit of the school of Cos under the leadership of Hippocrates.

The spirit of the oath is echoed in the ethical works ascribed to Hippocrates or his students. 'Regarding the art of medicine', he says in the work *On art*, 'I must first say what I believe its scope to be: to take away suffering or at least alleviate it. The fact that even those who do not believe in it can be cured by it is strong proof of its existence and power.'

Again, in the work *On the physician*, he says: 'For the physician it is undoubtedly an important recommendation to be of good appearance and well-fed, since people take the view that those who do not now how to look after their own bodies are in no position to look after those of others. He must know how and when to be silent, and to live an ordered life, as this greatly enhances

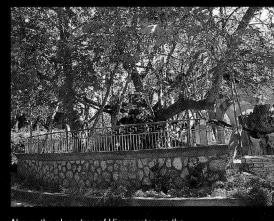

Above: the plane tree of Hippocrates on the island of Cos. Some lines from the Hippocratic Oath are quoted on the page opposite.

his reputation. His bearing must be that of an honest man, for this he must be towards all honest people, and kindly and understanding. He must not act impulsively or hastily; he must look calm, serene and never cross; on the other hand, it does not do for him to be too jolly.'

27...

The ethical works and the oath are part of the *Corpus Hippocraticum*; a group of medical treatises of various schools and epochs, which were collected in the third century BC for the library at Alexandria.

The fact that only a few of the works included in the famous *Corpus* are from Hippocrates himself is of no importance, since what matters is the man and his masterly system. In spite of all their contradicitons, they all share a naturalistic approach – being practical rather than theoretical.

According to his first biographer, Soranus of Ephesus, who wrote some time in the first and second centuries AD, Hippocrates was born on the island of Cos in 460 or 450 BC and was the son of a doctor. He learned medicine from his father and travelled widely; he is known to have visited Thessaly, Thrace and the Propontis, and he may have been as far afield as Libya and Egypt. For many years he taught in the school of Cos and, when he died, his fame was so great and the awe in which he was held so high, that it was widely believed that honey from the bees on his grave had extraordinary healing properties.

Hippocrates won his formidable reputation through his outstanding talent and ability. He had a profound understanding of human suffering, and put the doctor at the service of the patient, saying that his place was at the bedside of the sick. He showed how suffering could be alleviated not by any help from magic, but by hygiene and by proven cures. He set medicine on a new and historically decisive course, abandoning the gods for clinical observation.

Besides giving specific orientation to treatment, Hippocrates related all the medical knowledge of his age to a concept of disease which, as will be seen, weathered the test of time and survived to the beginning of the present era.

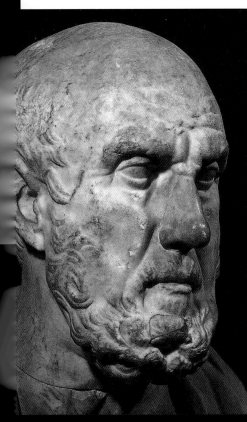

Above: Hippocrates, perhaps the greatest figure in the entire history of medicine.

Finally, he devised a method of diagnostic investigation based on observation and on reason which is valid today.

The weakness of Hippocratic teaching lay in its lack of anatomy and physiology, the very foundations of modern medicine. Contemporary knowledge of anatomy had to come from experiments on animals, since Greek respect for the dead meant that human dissection was banned. Again, Hippocratic medicine, fundamentally clinical and practical, focused wholly on the sick man and ignored the healthy person. The facts ascertained were therefore not adequate for building up into a substantial mass of background knowledge.

Hippocrates's followers believed that the body was formed from the union of the four elements, earth, air, fire and water, and the union of their attributes, that is, hot and cold, wet and dry. Innate heat was the basic condition of life, and when it failed death ensued. For this heat to be maintained at constant level, pneuma must penetrate the body through the windpipe and circulate in the veins with the blood.

If a concept of disease based on the harmony of the humours seems fantastic today, it was still regarded as valid in the first half of the nineteenth century. In fact, these concepts did not affect treatment, which as criteria of effectiveness used outside signs of disturbance, such as fever, inflammation, boils, abscesses and diarrhoea. These were thought of as timely and desirable means of purging, like any organic excretions. When body humours were in a state of imbalance, the aim of nature was to restore the situation to normal.

...28

The writings of the Hippocratic school give interesting information on the treatment of fractures and dislocations. These illustrations from the eleventh-century *Commentaries of Apollonius of Chitiron on the Peri arthron of Hippocrates* show, below, treatment for a dislocated jaw and, right, a method for reducing dislocated vertebrae.

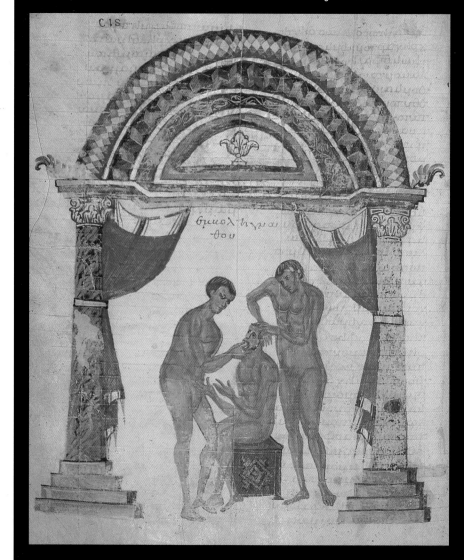

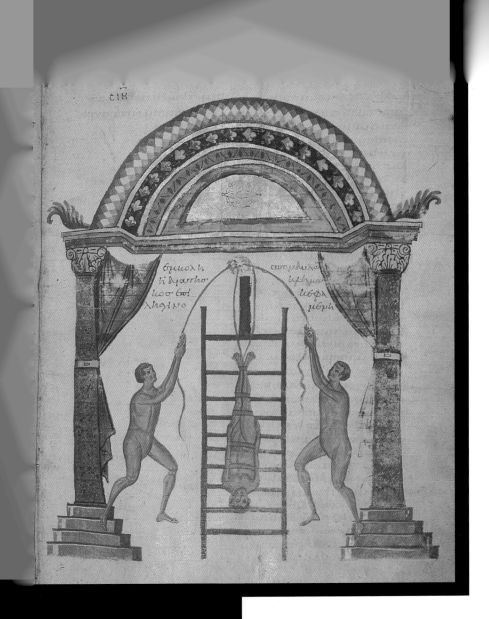

Hippocrates had a profound understanding of human suffering and emphasized that the place of the doctor was at the patient's bedside.

Constitutional pathology is of far greater interest from the modern point of view. It forms the subject of the book *On airs, waters and places,* one which can be attributed to Hippocrates with certainty. It represents the first real enquiry into the influence of external factors both on man's physical make-up and on the ethnological features of various racial types.

One of the main passages advises: 'Whoever intends to understand medicine aright must learn all that is written here. First he must consider the effect of each of the seasons of the year and the differences between them. He must take note of the winds, cold or warm, both those common to every country and those localized to one region. Lastly he must note the different qualities of water, varying in taste and in effects on the body . . . In the same way, he must observe how men live, what they like, what they eat and what they drink, whether or not they take physical exercise or are idle and gross. All this a doctor must know, in order to understand local complaints and be in a position where he can prescribe suitable treatments for them'.

The Hippocratic practitioner did his rounds before noon, 'because in the morning both patient and physician are in a more tranquil frame of mind.' Having enquired about what sort of night the patient had passed and how his bowels were functioning, the physician proceeded to a careful examination of the body, respiration, sweat and urine of the patient. The temperature was taken by laying a hand on the chest; percussion revealed how hard and large was the liver, and also gave information about the spleen and lungs. Next the physician performed auscultation, bearing in mind the master's invaluable advice. Hippocrates's descriptions were precise and to the point. Of an attack of pleurisy, for example, he says: 'when the lung touches the ribs and the patient coughs, there is pain in the thorax, and a sound is heard like leather rubbing against leather'.

Prognosis was highly important. Every change was carefully recorded. The facies Hippocratica, as it is still called, gave cause for serious alarm. 'Nose peaked, eyes sunken, temples hollow, ears cold and contracted with lobes turned outwards, sweat clammy, yellowish hue. . . .' This appearance signified impending death, as Shakespeare recognized; when Falstaff died, Mistress Pistol reported it in these words, '. . . for after I saw him fumble with the sheets, and play with flowers, and smile upon his fingers' end, I knew there was but one way: for his nose was as sharp as a pen. . . .' Besides the facies, some other prognostic signs are still linked with his name, such as Hippocratic succession, a splashing sound heard when pus is on the chest.

One of the chief glories of the Hippocratic *Corpus* lies in the case reports and aphorisms, which give a vivid illustration of the Greek genius for seizing on essential facts. The descriptions it gives of tuberculosis, typhus, mumps and malaria, among others, are classics. Hippocrates included these case histories from his three years' practice on the island of Thasos in the first of the seven books of *On epidemics*.

He gives a clear clinical picture of mumps: 'Some people had high fever, in most cases benign, and nose-bleeds. No one died. But many people suffered from swellings near the ears, sometimes on one side only but more often on both. Most had normal temperatures and stayed up and about. A few had slight fever. All the swellings disappeared and there were no harmful after-effects; in no case was there suppuration, as is usual with swellings occurring in other disorders. The lumps were soft and large, diffuse, not inflamed and not painful. They disappeared in all cases without any trouble. The complaint affected many children and young people and also adults in their prime, especially those given to gymnastics, but few women were affected. Many had a dry unproductive cough and a hoarse voice. At the onset in some cases, and later on in others, there were painful swellings of the testicles on one side or both.'

The day-to-day experience of Hippocrates is contained in the 406 sayings in the famous book of *Aphorisms*. It is surprising how many old sayings and household phrases came first from the lips of this physician, such as 'Extreme ills need extreme cures'.

The first aphorism is well known: 'The life so short, the art so long to learn, the chance soon gone, experience deceptive and judgment difficult', while the last one, which is believed to have very ancient origins, and which was responsible for much suffering until centuries later, is: 'Those diseases which medicines do not cure, the knife does; those which the knife cannot cure, fire can cure, but what fire cannot cure must be deemed incurable.'

The *Aphorisms* were translated into Latin before the sixth century and by about the mid-thirteenth century a large proportion had been assimilated into the popular rhymes of the Salerno medical school, which were repeated in every literate household of western Europe.

This is how Hippocrates describes the requirements for operations in the *Aphorisms*, in his clear, succinct style: 'Required in the operating theatre for operations are the patient, the assistants, the surgeon, his instruments, and light. The surgeon, whether standing or seated, must be in a good light and in an appropriate position for the particular operation; he can use natural or artificial light, direct or indirect'.

...30

The first aphorism is well known: 'The life so short, the art so long to learn, the chance soon gone, experience deceptive and judgment difficult'.

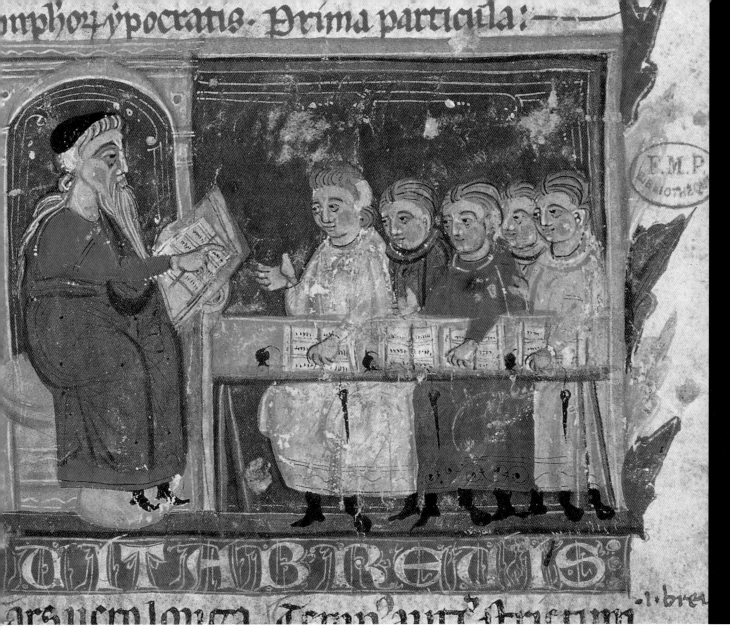

Above: an early manuscript illustration showing a teacher givng his pupils instruction on the aphorisms of Hippocrates.

Surgeons used bistouries and knives of various kinds, sounds of lead or bronze, straight or curving, the trepan for cranial operations, the cautery for haemorrhoids, the vaginal speculum for haemorrhage and fistulas, and the syringe and forceps for tooth extractions. The most fascinating section of the writings of the Hippocratic school on surgery deals with dislocations and fractures; bandaging and resting positions for fractured limbs are described carefully. To reset the femur, the patient was laid on a 'Hippocratic bench' with a windlass for control. The writer of the treatise concludes by saying: 'In short, it is like modelling in wax; the parts must all be put in their correct positions, whether they are badly aligned or abnormally joined together, adjusted by hand and bandaged in the same position; but the job must be done with a gentle touch, not roughly'.

Hippocrates believed that the body had the means of cure within itself, and the healing power of nature is often invoked in his works – 'Nature is the doctor' and 'Nature finds the way on its own' (*On epidemics*) and 'Nature acts without doctors' (*On diet*). His rational medical practice owed its greatness to this belief as well as to its encouragement of observation and experience and its avoidance of superstition and magic.

But almost immediately after the death of Hippocrates the school of Cos began to decline. The master's followers were not his equals and respect for his dicta was so great that no new contributions were forthcoming. Doctrines became ossified as dogma.

POST-HIPPOCRATIC MEDICINE

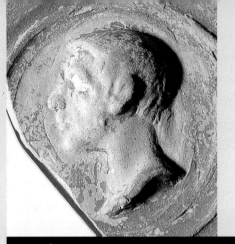

At the time of Hippocrates's death, Aristotle was a pupil of Plato in Athens. Later he was to be responsible for much original work on the fundamental problems of biology. Aristotle himself became tutor to Alexander, son of Philip of Macedon, who founded the town that bore his name. Alexandria became a new focus of Greek culture, with the most famous library of ancient times. At the medical school great advances were made in the neglected fields of anatomy and physiology, notably by Herophilus, who was said to have been the first man to practise human dissection and, incidentally, coined the words duodenum, meaning twelve digits long, and prostate. The school of Alexandria achieved much in the study of physiology and anatomy but no diplomas were given, however, with the result that many quacks and impostors capitalized on the fame of the school.

A great many Greek doctors, of varying ability, went to Rome, where Cato the Censor (234–149 BC), who admired only the austerity of the past, raged in the Senate against the effete way of life derived from Greece. He viewed Greek doctors with loathing; indeed, according to Pliny, he accused them of constituting a threat to Roman health. In a letter to his son Mark, Cato put him on his guard against the Greeks, a race of rogues, writing: 'If that pack pass on to us what they know, it will mean the end of Rome, especially if their doctors come here. For they have sworn death by medicine to barbarians, and the Romans are barbarians to them. Beware of doctors!' Unfortunately Cato had no plan of action against 'graeculi delirantes', the raving Greeks, as the Romans nicknamed them. The only cures he could offer were magic words, and cabbages, cooked and raw, which were his universal remedy.

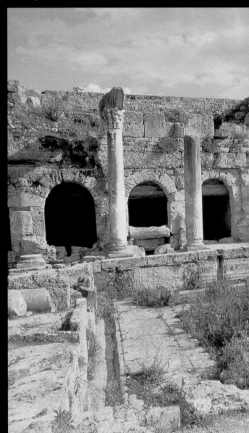

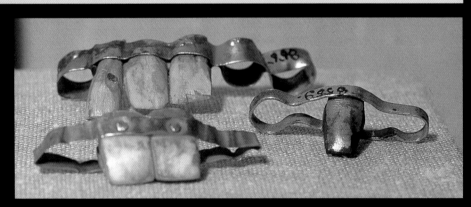

Top: Cato the Censor, a powerful reactionary who detested everything Greek.

Above: the Roman baths at Corinth, in Greece.

Left: Etruscan false teeth. The Etruscans were skilled dentists who devised methods of mounting extracted teeth on gold bridges.

Comparatively little is known about the Etruscans, who preceded the Romans, although undoubtedly they possessed some knowledge of medicine. Theophrastus remarks in his *History of plants* how 'Aeschylus in his elegies says Etruria is a land rich in remedies and that the Etruscan race make medicine'. Etruscan priests would have served as doctors to the Romans, who considered the practice of medicine ignoble. In the ruins of their temples, in fact, votive tablets representing organs of the human body and resembling those unearthed in the Aesculapian sanctuaries have been found. Dental crowns and gold fillings have also been unearthed and show the skill of Etruscan dentists. The Etruscans cultivated the ancient art of divination from the viscera of animals, especially the liver – in fact the word haruspex (soothsayer) comes from the Chaldean *har*, which means liver. From the Etruscans the Romans inherited knowledge of the therapeutic properties of certain waters and of building for public health purposes. The Cloaca Maxima or great drain was finished under the rule of Tarquinius Priscus in the sixth century BC. It drained stagnant water from marshy ground and emptied it into the Tiber; it was later adapted for sewerage, in the modern sense. The first aqueduct bringing a water supply into the city was built later and completed in 312 BC.

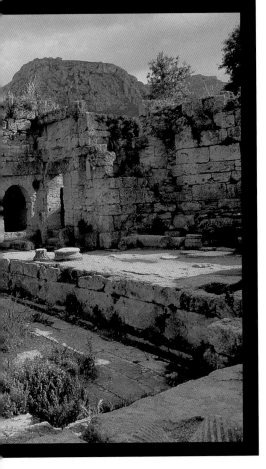

Asclepiades

It is clear that in the earliest times Roman medicine must have been both magical and supernatural, with various gods being responsible for the protection of health. The Romans were at first too proud to practise medicine, but they learnt that in Greece the profession of medicine was respected and entailed rigorous training at a recognized school, and so, later, they changed their views and master physicians began to arrive in increasing numbers.

Asclepiades of Prusa who had studied at Alexandria was the first Greek doctor to succeed in Rome. A man of great insight, he knew what would captivate the gluttons of Rome, spoiled by their wealth and oblivious of the uncomfortable austerity preached by Cato. It was useless to prescribe foul-tasting medicines; indeed, he did not even believe they worked. Instead, he prescribed diet, exercise, walking, baths and massage.

According to Celsus, Asclepiades, was 'in the forefront of doctors, and apart from Hippocrates the foremost', but Galen disliked his refutation of the Hippocratic theory of humours. The pathology of Asclepiades was based on the concept of the body as made up of atoms, elementary corpuscles imperceptible to the senses and continually moving through the pores and canals of the body. If liquid substances flowed through the cavities of the body without meeting obstacles, the body was in a state of health. Illness resulted if the circulation of liquids was impeded through some obstruction caused by the corpuscles. The obstacles could arise out of mass, number or anomalous movement of the atoms. Themison of Laodicea, a pupil of Asclepiades, added that illness, besides arising from the quality and movement of corpuscles, also occurred when the pores through which the atoms moved were unduly restricted or relaxed – diseases were thus of two types: those with a state of tension and those with a state of relaxation.

For this reason the Methodist school, following Asclepiades, laid great stress on taking baths to induce sweating when the pores were restricted and astringents and tonics when they were dilated. The Methodists held that illness could also be of a mixed type, in which case treatment of the dominant pathogenic factor was advised. Asclepiades did not share the faith of Hippocrates and his school in the healing powers of nature. Indeed, he believed doctors should act '*cito, tute et iucunde*' – in a fast, safe and pleasant manner. His material contributions to medicine include distinguishing between acute and chronic diseases and observing the periodicity of some diseases. Asclepiades described malarial fevers with accuracy; he was the first to carry out tracheotomy, probably for diphtheria; and he introduced humane methods in the treatment of the mentally deranged, transferring them from dark places, where they were usually hidden away, to well-lit buildings, where they carried out therapeutic exercises.

33...

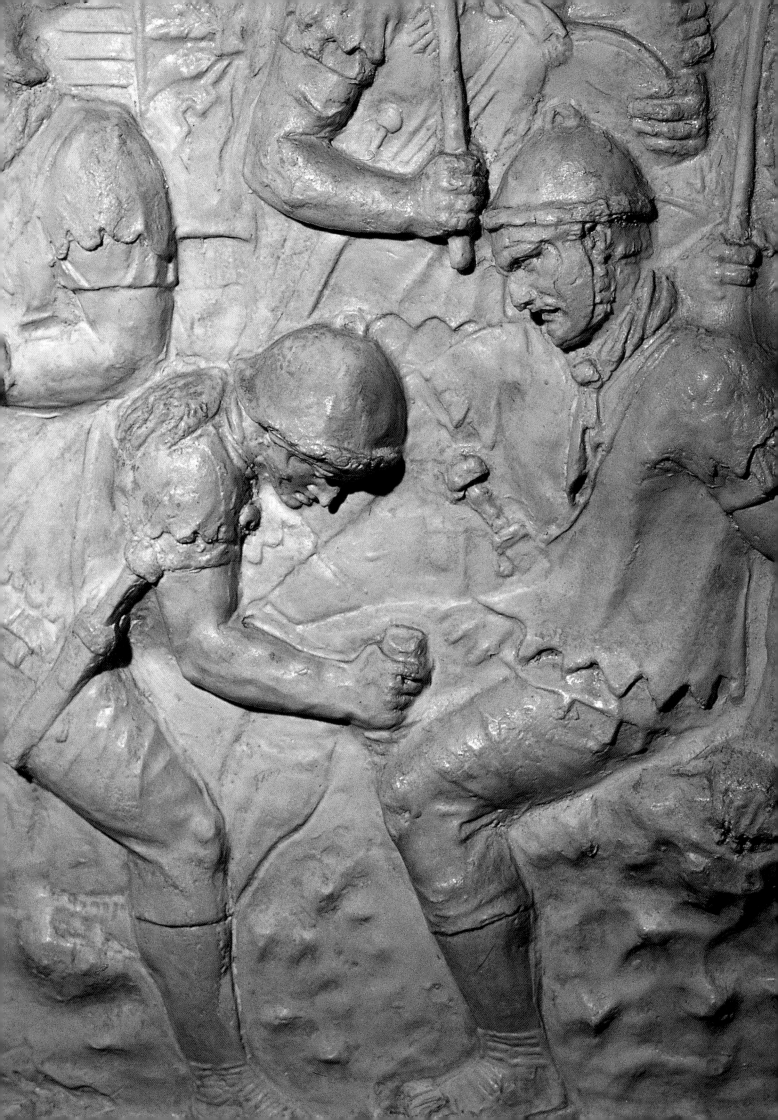

CELSUS AND PLINY, THE MEDICAL ENCYCLOPAEDISTS

Aulus Cornelius Celsus, who lived at the start of the Christian era, was the most famous of all Roman medical writers. His great encyclopaedic work, *De artibus*, embraced agriculture, military theory, philosophy and law, as well as medicine, the section on which, *De re medica*, is the only one to survive. Little known when it was written and forgotten in the Middle Ages, it was discovered in 1426 and, in 1478, became the first ancient text on medicine to be printed.

In this work Celsus avoided doctrinal disputes and arranged material systematically, subdividing diseases by treatment, which might be by diet, drugs or surgery. Celsus may have been faithful to the Hippocratic concept of pathology but in this work, which represented the first attempt at producing a complete textbook of medicine, there was considerable advance over the viewpoint of the great Greek physician.

Much new information was to be found in *De re medica*. Celsus described nutrient enemas, and plastic surgery on the nose, lips and ears. He wrote at length on the care of wounds and advised the use of compresses to stop bleeding and exerting pressure on and tying blood vessels. He understood the complications of wounds: 'Let nothing be undertaken until the inside of the wound has been cleaned, lest any congealed blood remain within it. For this will turn to pus and cause inflammation which will prevent the wound from healing'. Lastly, the edges of the wound were to be sewn up with thread or better still held together by means of clips. Celsus stated the four cardinal signs of inflammation – '*rubor, calor, dolor, tomor*' (redness, heat, pain, swelling) – which are still memorized today by every medical student.

Treatment for broken bones is clearly set out. First the fracture was

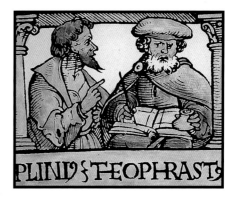

Above: Pliny, the Roman naturalist, with Theophrastus, a celebrated botanist and pupil of Aristotle.

Left: a doctor tends a wounded soldier. A bas-relief showing an incident during Trajan's war with the Dacians. From Trajan's Column, Rome.

35...

Celsus's *De re medica*, the only part to survive of his vast compendium of knowledge, is the earliest scientific medical work in Latin.

reduced, and then immobilization of the affected part was achieved by splints and bandaging, stiffened by wax and flour paste; the bandages were to be changed after one week or at most nine days, when the swelling had gone down. For open fractures, Celsus advised resection of the protruding fragment. For abdominal lesions, he suggested sewing up the large intestine, but excluded all possibility of effective treatment for lesions of the small intestine.

Surgical instruments found during archaeological excavations at Pompeii, now in Naples national museum, fit his descriptions exactly. Besides various types of forceps, scalpels, hooks, sounds, probes and tongs, there were ingenious devices new to the surgical armoury: one, called the meningophylax, was used after trephining the skull to hold back the meninges; another, like an iron V, was used to keep a wound open while removing an arrowhead; a lithotome was used for surgical removal of stones; and special forceps were employed to remove bone fragments after trephining.

Caius Plinius Secundus (AD 23–79) – Pliny the elder – was the greatest Roman naturalist and also an encyclopaedist, whose massive *Natural history*, a work in thirty-seven books, revealed a wealth of scholarship. Pliny, like Cato the censor, disliked physicians, but his work is of interest from the medical standpoint since he dealt with drugs obtainable from vegetable, animal and mineral sources, and gave many references to public health in his time and to names and events which would otherwise be unknown to us.

Right: a Roman forceps of the type in use during
Soranus's time.

Far right: a birth scene showing delivery with a
midwife. From the tomb of Scribonia Attice
Amerimno, in the Isola sacra burial ground, Ostia.

SORANUS, FATHER OF OBSTETRICS AND GYNAECOLOGY

...36

In Roman times, both magic and the skill of midwives were of importance in childbirth. The ancients had devised Caesarean section, but used it only on the dead or dying woman, and knew of no other obstetrical procedures, partly because the anatomical ideas of the Hippocratic school about genital organs were incomplete. With vague notions of anatomy, their ideas about the physiology of fertilization were also hazy. They knew, however, about the different positions of the foetus and how some of these made delivery difficult.

The first great obstetrician in history was Soranus of Ephesus (AD 98–138). A member of the Methodist school, he practised medicine at Alexandria before settling in Rome and is today regarded as the father of obstetrics. His main work, *On the diseases of women*, was a textbook which remained in use for fifteen centuries. In it, he described the female genital system in detail and likened the uterus to a cupping instrument open during coitus and menstruation. He advised contraception by means of cotton, ointments or fatty substances, but disapproved of abortion by mechanical means. He also described menstruation, conception and amenorrhoea, which could have physiological causes, such as child-bearing and breast-feeding, or pathological causes, such as inflammation of the genital tract or debilitating disease, and he prescribed treatment for uterine bleeding and for dysmenorrhoea.

He dealt with the difficulties that could attend childbirth and then, having taken care of the mother, Soranus went on to describe the care, health and growth of the newborn child. Breast-feeding was not to start until the third day; on the first two days, the baby was to be fed on honey, diluted and boiled. He also suggested what to do if the mother's milk failed, and gave advice on weaning, teething and teaching infants to walk. Finally, he gave some account of childhood diseases, and how to avoid and how to treat them.

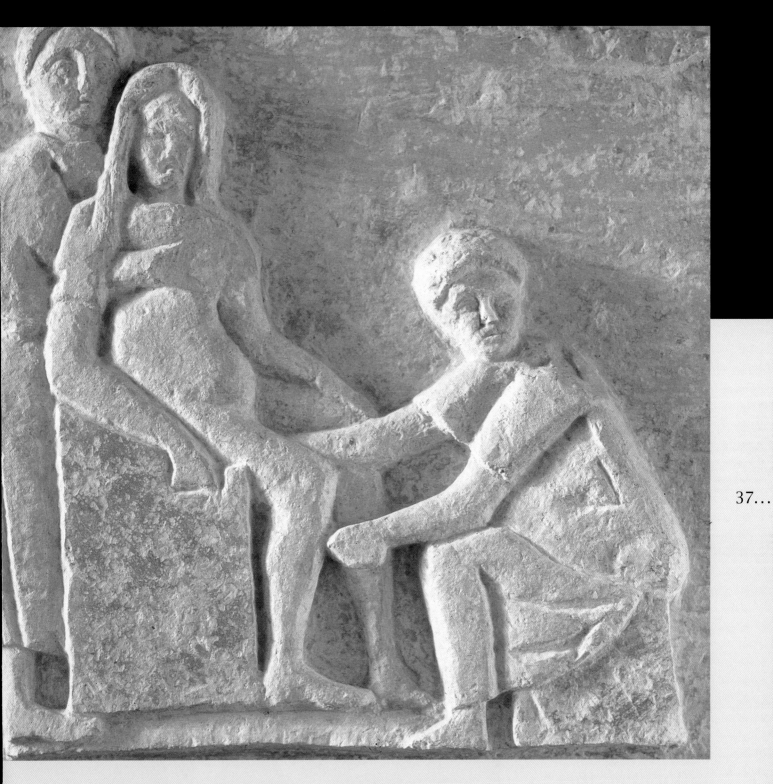

Soranus of Ephesus, who lived in the first century, was the most famous obstetrician of ancient times and the author of *On the diseases of women*, a text which remained in use for fifteen centuries.

As well as childcare, Soranus also wrote treatises on acute and chronic diseases and on fractures. His works were plagiarized in succeeding centuries by writers who went so far as to claim authorship of them.

Just as the writings of Soranus remained a standard text on obstetrics and gynaecology for centuries, so the work of Dioscorides was used as a textbook in pharmacology until the Renaissance. Born about AD 40, Dioscorides became one of the best known and respected army surgeons at the time of the emperor Nero. His chief work, *Materia medica*, in five books, contained all the pharmacological information available under the Roman empire, with an appendix on poisons and antidotes. The first book of *Materia medica* was devoted to herbs, ointments and oils; the second to food products from animals such as honey and milk, and from agriculture such as wheat; the third and fourth books dealt with plants and roots; the fifth with wines, and medicines from the mineral

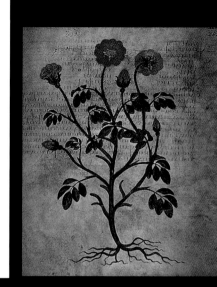

...38 Dioscorides was an army surgeon whose *Materia medica* described over six hundred medicinal plants and has deeply influenced the modern pharmacopoeia.

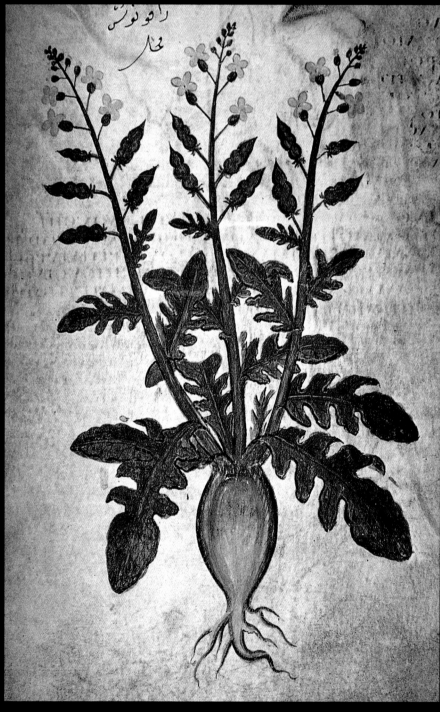

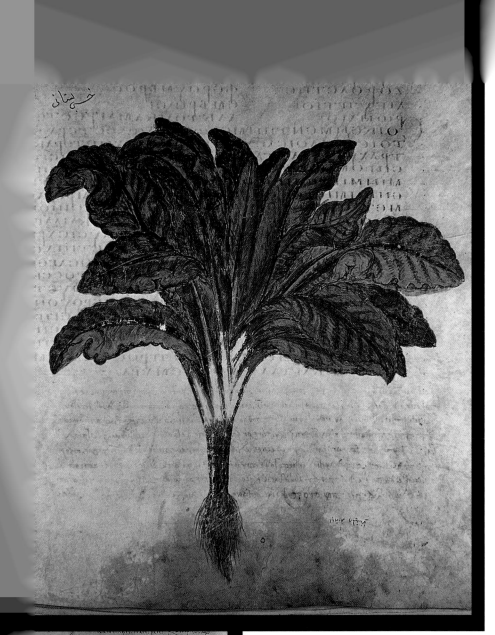

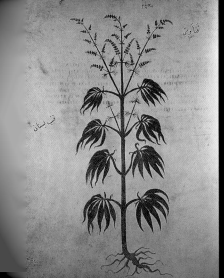

Above: Four medicinal plants described by Discorides, from an early manuscript. Clockwise from top right, lettuce, opium poppy, rhubarb and the rose.

kingdom such as lead acetate, copper oxide and calcium hydroxide. The original Greek text was soon translated into Latin and illustrations were added; many copies of these versions have come down to us from a ninth- or tenth-century codex dedicated to a Byzantine princess, Juliana Anicia.

At this time there were doctors of many kinds practising in the Empire, from those who treated slaves to the court doctors and the highest of all, the Palatine doctor. In addition there were doctors for the poor, employed by municipalities, and doctors to the army and the gladiators. In a similar way, there were also several kinds of hospitals, some caring for slaves, some for athletes and gladiators, and others for the military. As the Roman Empire declined the status of the doctors increased. Physicians became more and more respectable and respected: instruction in medicine became systematized and at the same time the political power of doctors emerged and was increasingly felt, so that by the time of the later emperors the physicians were often the most important members of the court and the trusted friends of the ruler.

Although the Roman doctors did not excel as theoreticians their laws for hygienic regulation of baths and aqueducts were exemplary; the system of drains and canals was properly supervised; conditions for food sales in the market places were subject to certain controls; and orders were in force in respect of the burial and cremation of the dead, so they could be said greatly to have advanced public health.

Right: the title page of an edition of Galen's collected works published in Venice in 1586.

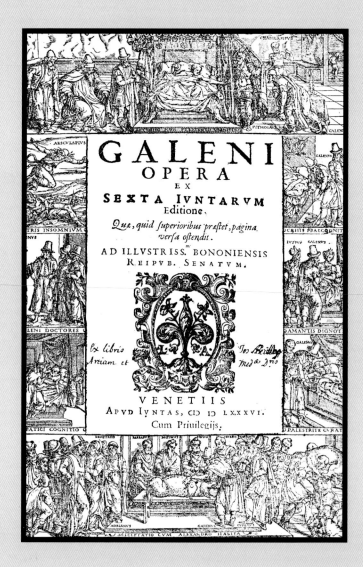

GALEN

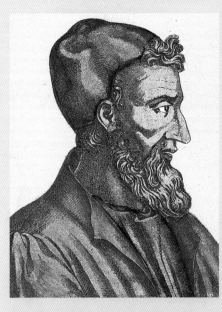

Above: an imaginary portrait of Galen, probably dating from the the fifteenth century.

Claudius Galen is a giant in the annals of medicine. Without the bias of post-Hippocratic schools, yet loyal to the teaching of the master of Cos, Galen summarized and systematized all the medical knowledge of ancient times, with reasoning that was always based on observation and experience. The first printed edition of his work filled twenty-two massive volumes, equivalent to approximately one half the bulk of extant Greek and Roman medical literature. Together with the *Corpus Hippocraticum*, it represents the sum of medical achievement in antiquity.

Galen was born at Pergamon in Greece in about AD 130, and studied at Smyrna and Alexandria. In the year 162 he went to Rome where he soon earned a reputation as a skilled medical practitioner and writer, becoming the physician and confidant of two emperors, Marcus Aurelius and Lucius Verus, as well as building up an enormous practice. What personality defect he suffered from is hard to guess, but he certainly had one, for he was always attacking his colleagues, suggesting that they were inept and that his own therapeutic and diagnostic ability was unparalleled.

Galen wrote some four hundred treatises, most of which were lost in a fire. Eighty-three were saved and are known to be genuine, because he was prudent enough to make a list. This great and most industrious of doctors employed a whole team of scribes to write down his every dictum. His thoughts on anatomy, mostly contained in the sixteen books of the work *On anatomical preparations,* were drawn from studies of the human skeleton, from his experience as surgeon to the gladiators and also from dissection of animals, but were marred by false deductions, since he applied to man what he learned from animals. Thus Galen found the rete mirabilis in the brain of a calf and assigned to this structure a vital physiological function in man – who does not possess it. Galen's descriptions of bones were admirable, his work on muscles accurate and he described in minute detail the brain, nerves and vascular system.

Galen's work on anatomy was impressive and contained the seeds of rapid progress, which might have been achieved if only students of the Middle Ages had thought to verify his findings. No checking was done, since dissection of human corpses was forbidden by the Christians and the Arabs, and so his observations stood unchallenged until the Renaissance and the revival of anatomy.

Galen's genius was evident in experiments conducted on animals for physiological purposes. The work *On the use of the parts of the human body* comprised seventeen books on this topic. To study the function of the kidneys in producing urine, he tied the ureters and observed swelling of the kidneys. To study the function of nerves, he cut them, and thereby showed paralysis of shoulder muscles after division of nerves in the neck and loss of voice after interruption of the recurrent laryngeal nerve. He also produced cardiac arrest by cutting the nerves to the heart and so finally dispelled the ancient misconception that nerves come from the heart rather than from the brain. He declared that every change in function of the body results from some kind of injury and that every injury leads to a change in function. This concept remains substantially valid.

41...

The fundamental principle of life, in Galenic physiology, was pneuma, which took three forms and had three types of action: animal spirit (pneuma psychicon) in the brain, centre of sensory perceptions and movement; vital spirit (pneuma zoticon) centring on the heart regulated the flow of blood and body temperature; natural spirit (pneuma physicon) resided in the liver, centre of nutrition and metabolism. Pneuma entered the body through the arteria aspera, that is the trachea, passed to the lungs and thence through the arteria venalis (the pulmonary vein) to the left ventricle, where it met the blood from the liver. In the liver, blood was impregnated with pneuma physicon and received, through the vena porta, the nutritive substances which the intestine had transformed into chyle. The blood was distributed from the liver to the veins, which ran from it like arteries from the heart. Through the vena cava, blood entered the heart on the right side.

Blood was held in the right ventricle for a while to free it of impurities, which were then expelled from the lungs with the breath. But a small amount of blood passed from the right to the left ventricle through minute, invisible pores in the interventricular septum. The intake of vital spirit was then distributed to the whole body through the arterial system, some of it reaching the brain where it split into the intricate network of the rete mirabilis already mentioned. In the brain, vital spirit was transformed into animal spirit and distributed throughout the body by means of the nerves, which Galen envisaged as empty ducts.

Galen was therefore convinced that the venous and arterial systems were each sealed and separate from each other. William Harvey, who discoverered the circulation of the blood, wondered how Galen, having got so close to the answer, did not arrive at the concept of the circulation.

> Galen declared that every change in function of the body results from some kind of injury and that every injury leads to a change in function.

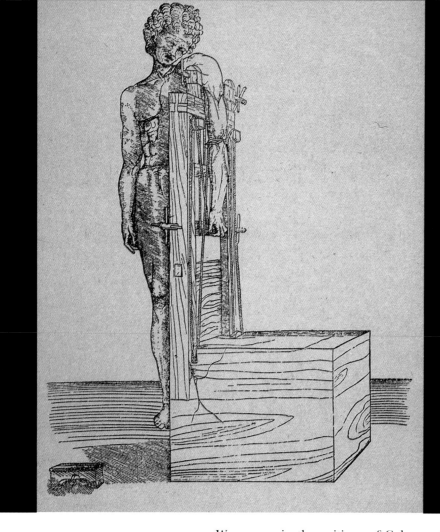

Left: treatment for a dislocated shoulder. From a sixteenth-century edition of Galen's works.

Below right: Galen (left) with Hippocrates. A thirteenth-century fresco from a church in Latium, 1231.

Galen's work, both his important discoveries and his false assumptions, was to remain unchallenged for over a thousand years.

We possess in the writings of Galen and others numerous testimonies to his diagnostic acumen and therapeutic skill, as well as his considerable anatomical knowledge. One of his cures, a typical example of his methods, created a great stir in Rome:

A Persian lost sensation in the ring and little fingers and half of the middle finger of one hand. He first called in some physicians, who tried emollients and then astringents without success, and then consulted Galen, whose first question was 'Have you been injured in the arm?' The Persian replied that he had fallen on a sharp stone and had suffered a hard blow between the shoulders with the immediate onset of a violent pain which rapidly decreased. Galen diagnosed a lesion of the spinal cord and prescribed rest in bed with soothing applications to the upper part of the back, and the patient recovered. Afterwards Galen explained that he had thought the source of the trouble was the region of the seventh (lowest) vertebra of the neck because he knew that every nerve had a distinct origin from every other nerve, even though nerves bunched together to form plexuses, and that the ulnar nerve, which carried sensation from the affected fingers, came from the spine at the level of the seventh cervical vertebra. He added that there was subsequently a heated controversy among physicians over the reason for the loss of sensation without loss of power in the involved part of the hand; Galen maintained that there were separate nerves for the skin and for the muscles, and that damage to the former had occurred in the Persian without the latter being affected.

Galen's diagnostic supremacy lay partly in his recognition of physical signs, some of which he showed to be characteristic of specific conditions. Time and again he impresses by the acuteness of his observations, as when he notes that the escape of air from a chest wound indicates that the lung has been pierced, and when he distinguishes accurately between bleeding from the kidneys and from the bladder by the appearance of the urine.

The treatments employed by Galen were derived from the concept of 'contraria contrariis' – the therapy of opposites – and so he applied heat if disease resulted from cold and purgatives for conditions where the body was thought to be over-burdened. In addition to diet and drugs, some of which were thought to have specific effects and indications, Galen also made great use of physiotherapy and other ancillary measures.

Why then did Galen, for all his mistakes, remain an unchallenged and unchallengeable authority for over a thousand years? How was it that after he died in 203, serious anatomical and physiological research ground to a halt, because everything there was to be said on the subject had been said by Galen? Although he was not a Christian Galen believed in one god, and declared that the body was an instrument of the soul. This made him most acceptable to the fathers of the Church and to Arab and Hebrew scholars. Since God did nothing by chance, there must be a relation between cause and event. Animated by this doctrine of final causes, he sought the why and the wherefore of everything; his explanations made it look as though he had all the answers. Yet this man, whose authority and mistakes perpetuated fundamental errors for nearly fifteen hundred years, was a physician, observer and experimenter of so high an order that today it is impossible not to regard him with esteem.

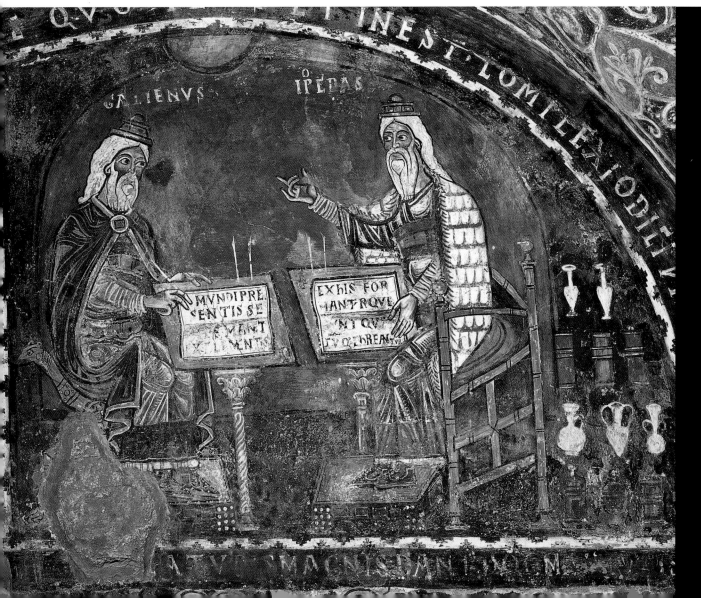

THE
DECLINE OF ROME

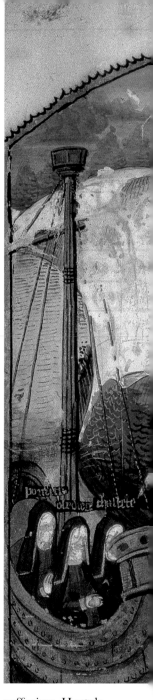

Galen wrote when the Roman Empire was at its zenith, but his works, which synthesized all the scientific thought of the ancient world, marked the beginning of a long decline in medical science.

Some of the reasons for the break-up of the empire – private and public corruption, oppression of minorities and widespread poverty, and the attacks by the barbarians on Roman territory – obviously relate to what happened to medicine, for under such conditions rational, objective thought would have been impossible. Another cause, the epidemics and plagues that ravaged the empire, involved doctors directly; and, as happened in Europe in the Middle Ages, the powerlessness of medicine to do anything but observe the pestilence carried people away from science and reason.

In many of the outbreaks of what was described as plague by several of the ancient writers, the only common characteristic was a high death rate. The physical features of a number of different diseases seem to be recorded; there are descriptions of blisters and pustules, erythema and pallor, haemorrhages and asphyxia, for smallpox, bubonic plague, scarlet fever, cholera, exanthematous typhus and diphtheria were clearly all included under the general heading of plague.

Historical circumstances had prepared the way for a rise of the mystical element of Christianity, the religion which offered brotherhood and charity to the humble and the afflicted, and gave consummate meaning to earthly life. Bodily ills could only be cured with divine aid, as was demonstrated in the gospel accounts of miraculous healing by Jesus, achieved by invoking the help of God the Father. Instead of medicaments, use was made of anointing with holy oil, prayer and the laying on of hands. Christianity, following the teaching of the Lord, regarded medicine as a work of charity. Religion reaped untold advantage from having instilled the idea of helping the sick as a bounden duty, from which neither the individual nor the community was exempt.

In practical terms, the Christians did much to relieve suffering. Hostels were built to shelter pilgrims and in time became proper hospitals. The first great Christian hospital was built by St Basil at Caesarea in the year 370 and the first hospital in the western world was built in Rome about 400. Although medical practice and surgery in particular continued to show signs of appreciable progress at this time, the figure of the lay doctor was on the decline, for the church viewed the care of the sick as a moral obligation incumbent on its members, and as a calling rather than as a paid profession.

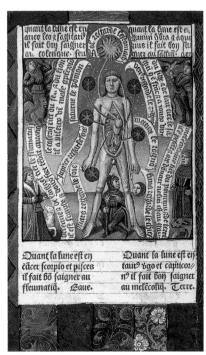

Above: an illustration from a mediaeval manuscript showing the great Paris hospital, the Hôtel-Dieu. On the left a novice is arriving to join the Augustinian sisters while, on the right, a patient is carried in on a stretcher.

Left: The Anatomy of Man, from a mediaeval miniature. According to a theory which dated back to the time of Pythagoras, there are four principle humours in the human body; phlegm, blood, choler (melancholy) and bile, the balance of which is essential for good health.

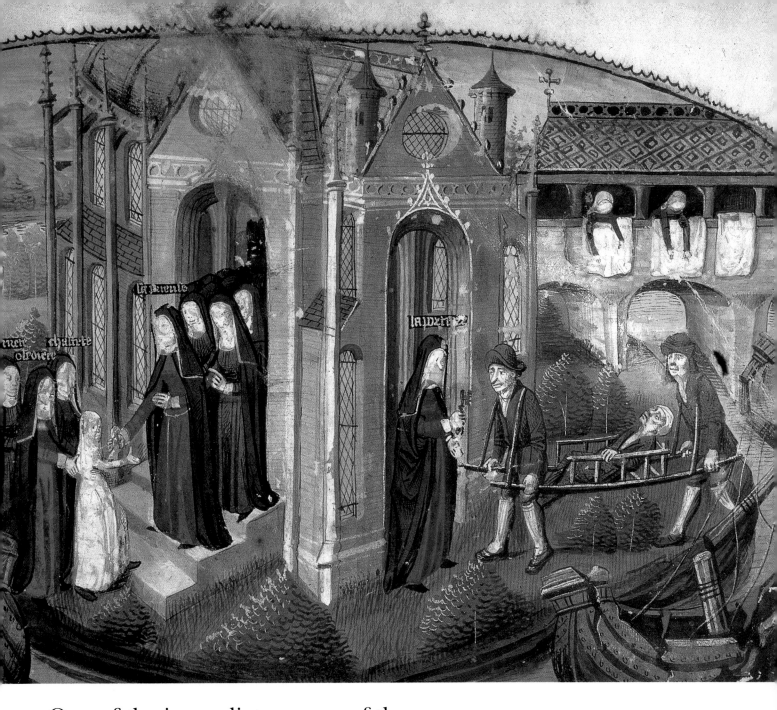

One of the immediate causes of the collapse of the Roman Empire was a series of epidemics and plagues. The doctors of the day were powerless in the face of these disasters, which led to an almost universal reaction against the scientific and rational approach to disease which was still slowly evolving, with a widespread resurgence of superstitious practice.

THE RISE
OF ARAB LEARNING

The Christian spirit of charity went so deep that it even pervaded a number of movements that had been declared heretical by the Church. The church founded by the Nestorian sect is an example. Expelled from the Empire, the Nestorians went to Persia where they founded the school of Gondishapur, which was to become the cradle of the Arab school of medicine. There (and at other sites in the Middle East) they built a great hospital, the staff of which became justly famous. The doctors of the Bukht-Yishu family were particularly highly regarded.

The first 250 years after the Hegira (Mahomet's flight to Medina on 16 July 622) saw the development of a young and vigorous Arab culture. In this period, medicine was led by the Bukht-Yishu family and by translators who rendered into Arabic the works of western medicine from Hippocrates to Galen. The new golden age of Hellenic culture came with the Abbasids who in a series of lightning campaigns within the space of a few years conquered not only the Middle East but Egypt, North Africa and Spain.

The first two Abbasid caliphs, Harun al-Rashid (763–809), who founded the first hospital in Baghdad, and his son al-Ma'mun (786–833) gave a great impetus to culture. Al-Ma'mun acquired many Greek manuscripts and built up a great library in Baghdad and numerous translations were made.

Many Arabic scientific terms have Greek or Syriac roots. On the other hand, many chemical terms of modern western civilization, such as alcohol, alkali, alkaloid, aldehyde, alchemy and alembic come from Arabic. The man who laid the basis of chemical science and devised the alembic or retort (in Arabic, al-*anbiq*) was Jabir ibn Hayan, who lived in the ninth century. Jabir may have been the first to make use of the procedures of filtration, sublimation and distillation; he was certainly the first to examine the blood and faeces.

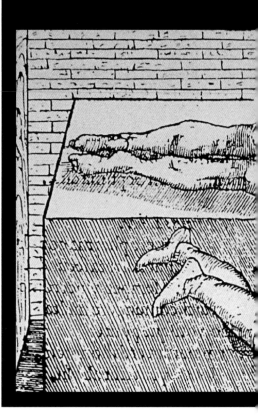

Avicenna's *Canon* had an enormous influence on medical teaching in the west as well as among the Arab-speaking peoples for many centuries.

Rhazes and Avicenna

The best known Arab medical writers were Rhazes and Avicenna, both associated with the eastern caliphate, and Avenzoar and Averroes who belonged to the school at Cordoba, the capital of the western caliphate. Abu Bakr Muhammad ibn Zakaria, known as al-Rhazes (860–932) was a Persian from near Teheran who studied medicine in Baghdad, where later he became established as the greatest Arab clinician of his time.

Rhazes was also interested in mathematics, astronomy, religion and philosophy; but over half of his 237 works treat of medicine. The most widely known were *al-Hawi*, known in the west as the *Liber continens*, an encyclopaedia of medical practice and treatment, and the *Liber medicinalis ad almansorem*, a compilation from various sources, but mainly from Hippocrates, Galen, Oribasius and Paul of Aegina, which contains such aphorisms as: 'When Galen and Aristotle agree about something, then it is easy for doctors to make a decision, but when they differ it is very difficult to arrive at agreement' and 'truth in medicine is an end that cannot be reached and all that is written in books is worth much less than the experience of a wise doctor'.

The treatise on smallpox and chicken-pox, the *Liber de pestilentia*, is his most important work, because it is entirely original and based on direct experience and observation, from which he drew very perceptive conclusions. Exact description was given of the clinical picture of both conditions, as well as information on differential diagnosis.

'The eruption of smallpox', wrote Rhazes, 'is preceded by continued fever, pains in the back, itching in the nose and delirium in sleep. Then acute prickling is felt and this goes all over the body, the cheeks go red and the eyes are inflamed. The patient has a sense of heaviness and general discomfort, he sneezes, yawns, feels pain in the throat and chest, and breathes and coughs

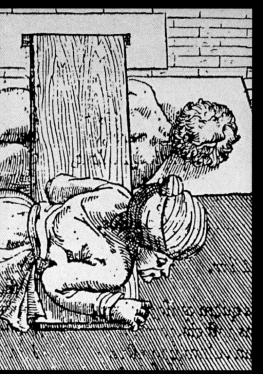

with difficulty. His mouth is dry and he has a headache, feels sick, restless and troubled. Note that feeling restless, sick and troubled is more frequent in chicken-pox, while pains in the back are features of the smallpox. Other signs are fever and marked reddening of the gums. When the pustules appear, care must be taken first of the eyes, then the nose and ears: very small white pustules coming up in contact with each other, hard and without fluid, are dangerous, and if the patient remains ill even after the eruption it is a fatal sign. When fever increases after the appearance of greenish or black pustules, and there is palpitation of the heart, it is a very bad sign indeed.'

Rhazes also had something to say about skin care, indicating how pustules could be prevented from leaving bad scars. Smallpox was known in antiquity, but Rhazes was the first to advocate a definite regime of treatment.

Abu Ali al-Husain ibn Abdallah ibn Sina, known to us as Avicenna, was the giant of this era of Arab learning, a polymath who captured the imagination of his own and later ages. Born in 980 at Afshena near Bukhara in Persia, Avicenna was a precocious boy. At sixteen, he began to study medicine, and by the age of eighteen he was already an experienced practitioner. He lived a turbulent existence and went through many vicissitudes, including imprisonment. Nevertheless, he managed to write many works on widely different subjects.

47...

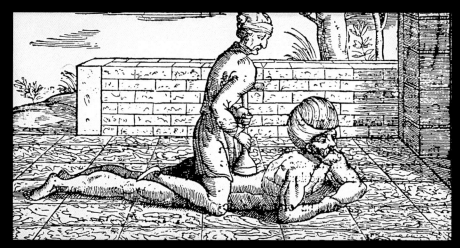

Above: illustrations from an early edition of Avicenna's *Canon*, showing treatment for a fracture or dislocation to the spinal column. In the top picture, pressure is being placed on the patient's back by using leverage on a board. In the lower picture, pressure is applied by pounding with a heavy instrument.

His masterpiece is the *al-Quanun* (the *Canon*) which served as a textbook in the medical schools of the western world for a considerable period. It represented an attempt on the grand scale to co-ordinate the medical doctrines of Hippocrates and Galen, and the biological ones of Aristotle. In the first of the five books of the *Canon*, Avicenna expounded the main doctrines of medicine, diseases and their symptoms, rules of health and hygiene, and also treatment. In the second book, largely based on Dioscorides, a series of medicaments were listed that were largely unknown to the Greeks. The third book dealt with pathology and contained recognizable accounts of pleurisy, jaundice, duodenal ulcer, pyloric stenosis and venereal diseases. The fourth book described the various contagious diseases, and included a treatise on surgery and a brief section on cosmetics, while the fifth book referred to the preparation of drugs and was the universally accepted text of *materia medica* up to the Renaissance.

The *Canon* was translated into Latin for the first time in the twelfth century by Gerard of Cremona. Together with the works of Galen, it dominated medical thinking in the Middle Ages. The main drawback of the Canon was inadequate basic anatomical and physiological knowledge; at times it seemed as if Avicenna was indulging in a private joke, for example when he analysed the nature of love and decided it was a mental disorder.

The lasting success of the *Canon* is most probably related to ideology, for Avicenna's idea was to reconcile the biological and medical doctrines of Aristotle and Galen, just as later Thomas Aquinas reconciled them with those of the Catholic church. The scholastic philosophy that was then elaborated by St Thomas to answer the attacks made on faith by reason recognized Avicenna and Averroes as masters who had transmitted the inheritance of Aristotle. This inheritance penetrated Spain and Sicily under the wing of Arab culture and thence to the rest of Europe, where Aristotle had been forgotten ever since the barbarians had served the links with the eastern empire.

Right: a doctor cauterizing leprous lesions. An illustration from *Chirurgia imperiale* (Imperial surgery), translated into Turkish from a treatise compiled in Persia during the thirteenth century.

...48

Below: helped by an assistant, an Arab doctor prepares a medicine. An illustration from a thirteenth-century manuscript.

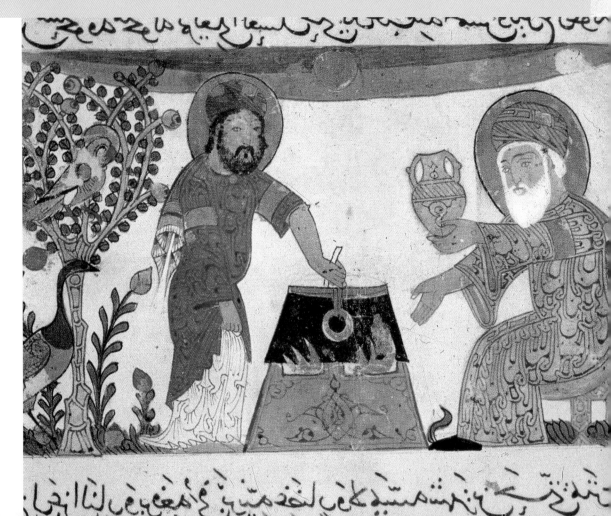

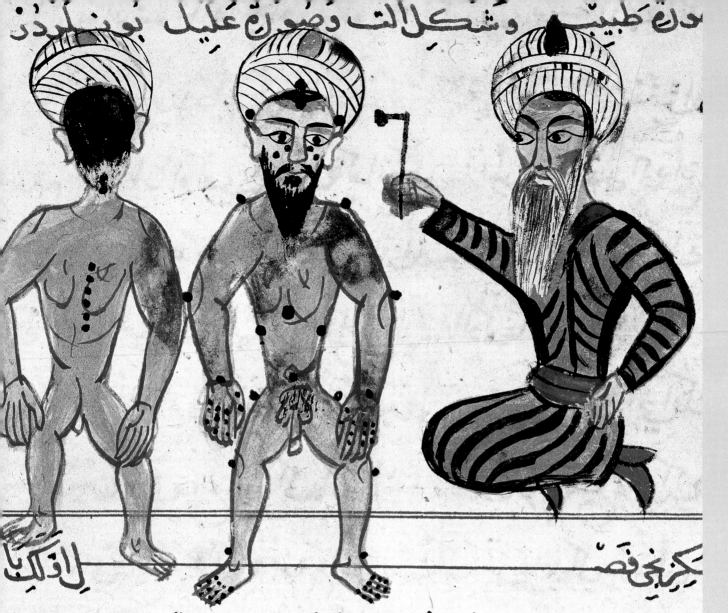

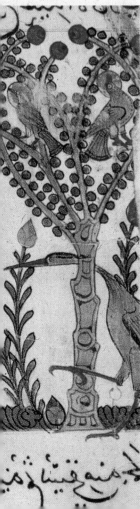

Avicenna was a polymath who captured the imagination of his own and later ages. A precocious child who could recite the entire Koran at the age of ten, he began to study medicine at sixteen and was an experienced practitioner at eighteen. However, although he read Aristotle's *Metaphysics* no less than forty times, he had to admit that, try as he might, he could not understand it at all.

When Avicenna died at the age of 57, the school of Cordoba was flourishing. In the tenth century, under the patronage of the great Caliph Abd al-Rahman III (912–961) of the Omayyad dynasty, the Spanish town became the leading cultural centre in Europe. It was full of doctors, and the welfare of the million or so inhabitants was assured by the fact that there were fifty-two hospitals.

Among this host of Cordoban doctors appeared the greatest surgeon of Islam, Abu'l-Quasim, Albucasis in the Latinized form. Little is known about his life apart from the fact that he was born in 936 at El Zahra near Cordoba. He left an encyclopaedic work entitled *al-Tasrif*, or the *Method*, translated into Latin by Gerard of Cremona, the most valuable part of which related to surgery. In fact, it contained observations which can be taken as revealing the hand of a highly skilled surgeon, and presented a mass of information on surgical practice at the time, with more than two hundred illustrations of the surgical instruments used by the Arabs.

Albucasis posed the question why Arab surgery was so far behind and concluded that this was due to insufficient knowledge of anatomy and of Galen, whom he obviously regarded highly. On surgical practice, he told surgeons, 'God is watching you and knows if you are operating because surgery is really necessary or merely for love of money.'

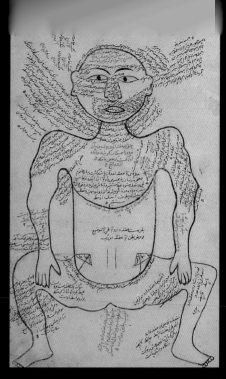

Three drawings from a fifteenth-century manuscript, *Tashrih al-badan* (Anatomy of the body), showing from the left, the muscular system, the digestive and arterial system and the skeletal system of the human body.

In the tenth century Cordoba became the cultural centre of Europe. The welfare of the million or so inhabitants was assured by the presence there of no fewer than fifty-two hospitals.

Cordoba

Under the Cordoban caliphate there was at least one non-conformist who was courageous enough not to accept the doctrines of the great men of the past without first evaluating them: this was Avenzoar, in Arabic Ibn Zuhr. He was born in Seville about the beginning of the twelfth century and died in 1162. As a doctor, he had no time for the metaphysical approach and placed great emphasis on practical experience. He therefore took a somewhat negative view of the *Canon* of Avicenna, while not even Galen was spared from his critical approach.

Ibn Rushid, or Averroes (1126–98), was better known as a philosopher than a doctor. He studied jurisprudence, philosophy and medicine and became a magistrate in Seville and Cordoba and later the governor of Andalucia. A heretic to both Moslems and Christians, he was nevertheless influential. His best known medical text is the *Colliget*, or *Collection*, an encyclopaedic work in the Galenic tradition, but which is more more concerned with the theory than the practice of medicine.

Averroes's most celebrated pupil was Musa ibn Maimun (1135–1204), better known as Maimonides, who was not an Arab but a Jew. He in turn followed Aristotle in trying to reconcile faith and reason. He refuted part of the rabbinical tradition, thereby arousing the hostility of orthodox fellow believers. Maimonides, like his master, became better known as a philosopher than as a doctor. Of special interest among his medical writings was the book of advice written for the depressive eldest son of the sultan Saladin, which contained dietetic and hygienic rules and served as an example to Italian writers on health and hygiene from the thirteenth to the fifteenth centuries.

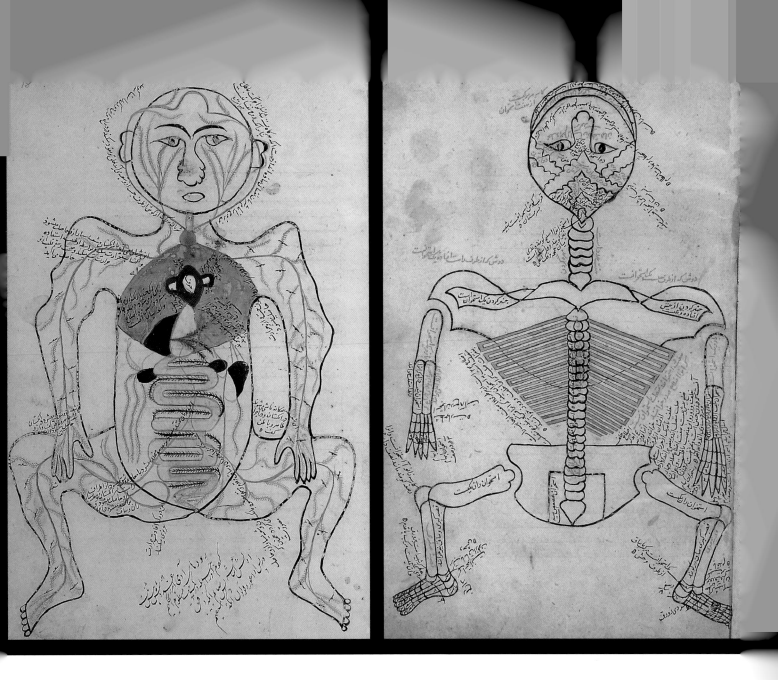

When Maimonides was thirteen, in 1148, the sect of Moslem fanatics called the Almohads displaced the Omayyads from Cordoba, which then declined rapidly. The Almohads determined to expel all the Jews and all the Christians who had not been converted to Islam. Maimonides fled with his family, lost everything in a shipwreck, and finally settled in Egypt, where he made a living from medicine, setting aside philosophy and the study of the Talmud. As a physician he was so famous that Richard Coeur de Lion offered him the post of personal physician, which he declined.

Twenty-eight years after Maimonides died, Cordoba was captured by Ferdinand II of Castile. Its culture had by then largely faded. The Moslems were gradually pushed out of Europe; in 1258, the Mongols destroyed Baghdad, and so after five centuries the Arab empire lay in ruins, its way of life lingering only as a memory. In the field of science and philosophy, the Arab heritage was a precious one. Medicine is indebted to the enlightened caliphs and their physicians who salvaged and treasured Greek traditions and Greek texts, and to the chemists who laid a scientific basis for pharmacology, and the legislators who recognized the continuing existence of the figure of the lay medical practitioner.

THE SCHOOL OF SALERNO

In the chaos which covered Europe in the early Middle Ages, the aftermath of successive wars, epidemics and famine, the welfare of the sick came into the hands of the religious orders, who were virtually the only people with sufficient detachment and peace to care for and comfort the sick, wounded and plague-stricken. At this time, every possible setback retarded the advance of medical investigation, and monastic peace was perhaps the one remaining hope.

St Benedict of Norcia did not set out to create a nursing order; chance circumstances were responsible for the progress of medicine, both in theory and in practice, in the hands of the Benedictine order. On the practical side, a number of monastic infirmaries were built. The best known of these belonged to the Swiss monastery of St Gall, which had been founded in 720 by an Irish monk. Monastic hospitals were entirely autonomous; medicines were made up by the monks themselves from plants grown in the herb garden.

Help was always readily available for the sick who came to the doors of the monastery. In time, the monks who devoted themselves to medicine emerged from their retreats and started visiting the sick in their own homes. This infringed the rules of the order by exposing the monks to the temptations of the world, and it became a hotly debated issue at ecclesiastical councils and synods. Eventually, monastic medicine was forbidden, but it wa church authorities to enforce this injunction. Many religiou name for themselves as healers and were in great demand; a ple, especially those who professed the faith, preferred their the lay doctors.

But lay medicine had not entirely disappeared, and aft period it came to the fore again and flourished in the famous This town had became a Roman colony in AD 194 and had health resort. The school of medicine gradually came into century and reached its height in the late eleventh century.

The first manual for the use of students, containing the and others was written about 1050 by Gariopontus, the most his time. The work was entitled the *Passionarius*, and is of va the basis of modern medical terminology. Gariopontus lati and took words from common speech, for example, cicatr Another text for students of the time was the *Practica* of Petro

The knowledge of the school of Salerno was mainly set o Another unusual feature of the school was in the presence o dents who are frequently referred to in the writings. Some name: '*ut ferrum magnes, juvenes sic attrahit Agnes*' (Agnes att iron to magnet).

One of the Salerno women was Trotula, who wrote *De n ante, in et post partum*, a treatise on obstetrics containing ad

Just as the Arabs collected and passed on the knowledge of the Greeks, so their own contributions were preserved in European medical thought, notably at Salerno.

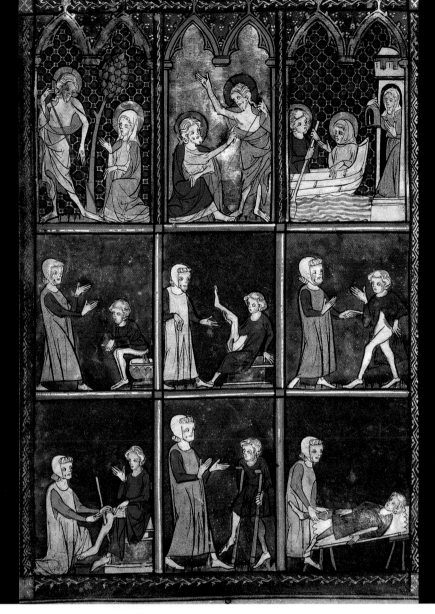

The knowledge of the school of Salerno was mainly recorded in light verse. Another particularly unusual feature of the school was the presence there of many female students.

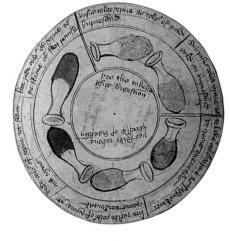

Above: a chart for the examination of urine, circa 1430. There were various systems of urinoscopy, giving details of colour, odour, etc., together with instructions for doctors on how to make a diagnosis. It was to remain an important diagnostic method for centuries.

before, during and after childbirth, on the treatment of prolapse and polyps of the womb, and on the choice of a wet nurse and her diet (an excess of highly salted foods, as well as garlic, onion and pepper was strictly forbidden). Trotula's identity is unknown; it has been suggested that she was not really a physician but a midwife, perhaps the wife of a famous doctor; another theory is that Trotula was a general nickname for all the Salernitan midwives. The treatise remained a standard text until the sixteenth century. This Salernitan character appeared in early English literature under the name Dame Trot, and later featured in Victorian books for children as Dame Trot with her cat.

The writings of the Salerno school were mostly collaborations, although the names of some individuals stand out. Rogerius Frugardi was the author of a clear and concise text on surgery, which however often echoed ideas and methods used by Greek doctors. The chapters on cranial and abdominal wounds are of particular interest. Fractures of the head should be explored by palpation, and in the case of depressed fractures he advised trephining a series of perforations so that the damaged bone could be removed without damage to the membranes covering the brain. In abdominal injuries, if the intestine had protruded for long enough to have turned cold and hard, Rogerius suggested that before replacing the intestine it should be warmed and softened by placing it over the intestines of a newly-killed animal. Then it was to be cleaned with a sponge and replaced in the abdomen, the wound being left open as long as the damage remained visible, after which a drain was to be inserted and the wound dressed every day.

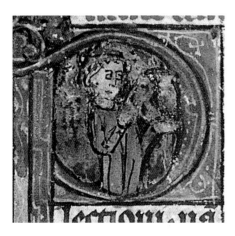

Above: Arnold of Villanova, one of the best-known physicians of the late thirteenth century who produced the first version of the *Regimen sanitatis Salernitanum*. He also acted for Spain on diplomatic missions and dabbled in alchemy.

...54

Doctors dissected animals, especially pigs, believing that there was a greater resemblance between human and pig intestines than between those of man and any other animal.

Salernitan anatomy was based predominantly on Galen. Doctors dissected animals, especially pigs, believing that there was more resemblance between human and pig intestines than between those of man and any other animals. A work by Copho belonging to the early period of the school was entitled *Anatomia porci* (Anatomy of the pig).

The Salernitan masters' idea of putting teaching matter into verse form was a happy inspiration. Their work, entitled the *Regimen sanitatis Salernitanum* (The Salerno book of health), provided the basis of clinical medicine up to the end of the Middle Ages. The great contribution made by the school was its popularization of practical medical knowledge in the form of aphorisms, in verse and with a spice of humour, which had a huge appeal.

The text was still in a phase of expansion when the first version was produced by Arnold of Villanova (1235–1315). This was printed for the first time in 1480 and had 362 verses, though they increased with time (a version with 3,520 verses was published later). The Regimen was dedicated to a king of England, who has remained unidentified, in these lines which are typical of the spirit of the work. This translation is by Sir John Harington, a godson of Queen Elizabeth I and was first published in 1607. Harington was also the author of

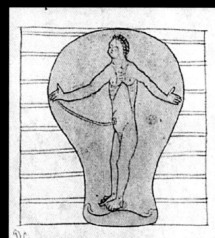
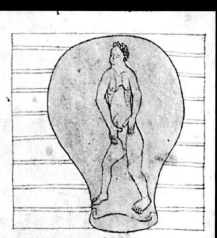
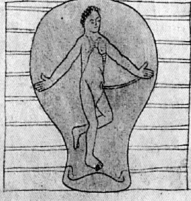
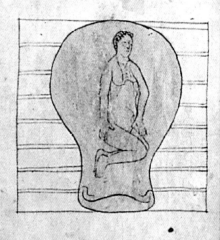

Salerno became Europe's first officially recognized medical school in 1224, when Frederick II made it an essential condition that anyone practising medicine in the kingdom of Naples must first seek approval from the masters of Salerno.

Left: a page from a late thirteenth-century English manuscript on obstetrics showing various positions of the foetus in the womb and giving advice on how to deal with complications.

The Anatomy of Ajax, 1596, describing his invention, the first flushing lavatory of modern times, and a translator of *Orlando Furioso*.

> The Salerno Schoole doth by these lines impart
> All health to Englands King, and doth advise
> From care his head to keepe, from wrath his heart,
> Drinke not much wine, sup light, and soone arise
> When meate is gone, long sitting breedeth smart:
> And after-noone still waking keep your eyes.
> When mou'd you find your selfe to Natures Needs,
> Forbeare them not, for that much danger breeds,
> Use three Physicians still; first Doctor quiet,
> Next Doctor Merry-man and Doctor Dyet.

This straightforward advice continues in a similar vein:

> Rise early in the morne, and straight remember,
> With water cold to wash your hands and eyes,
> In gentle fashion retching euery member,
> And to refresh your braine when as you rise,
> In heat, in cold, in July and December.
> Both comb your head, and rub your teeth likewise:
> If bled you haue, keep coole, if bath'd, keepe warme
> If din'd, to stand or walke will do no harme.

This poem went all over the known world; it was a huge success and was translated many times – there were versions in French, German, English and Italian. Official recognition for the school came in 1224, when an enactment of Frederick II made it obligatory for anyone practising medicine in the kingdom of Naples to seek approval from the masters of Salerno. Subsequently the school declined, for competition increased as universities sprung up in many other places. Culture, which had flourished on the shores of the Mediterranean, began to move northwards.

55...

The school of Salerno did not teach other subjects besides medicine and did not evolve into a *studium generale* as the universities founded in western Europe at that time were called. The universities began to grow up in the twelfth and thirteenth centuries. Their foundation, one of the most important events in the history of civilization, was made possible by the growth and increasing wealth of mediaeval cities.

One of the greatest of the ancient universities was Bologna, where a law school had been in existence since the eleventh century. One of the first teachers of medicine was Thaddeus of Florence (1223–1303), who is mentioned by Dante, who probably attended his lectures, whose highly priced professional services were also in great demand. He translated Aristotle and wrote a work, *Della conservazione della salute* (How to stay healthy), which recommended daily exercises. Another of his works is the *Consilia*, which described clinical cases in Italian rather than Latin.

The dissection of the dead is known to have been practised at Bologna at this time, initially under orders from the magistrature. In 1302, a nobleman called Azzolini met his death in suspicious circumstances. Doctor Bartolomeo da Varignana was instructed to examine the corpse and find out if death had been due to poisoning. He performed the autopsy and his report suggests a considerable practical knowledge of anatomy.

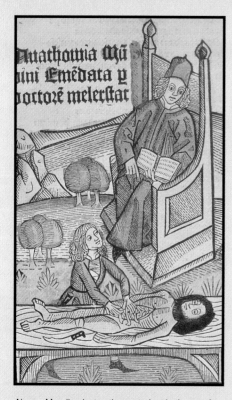

Above: Mondino instructing a student in the art of dissection, an illustration from his *Anathomia*, regarded as one of the most valuable of anatomical texts until the end of the sixteenth century.

Mondino

Anatomy took on a new lease of life in the hands of Remondino de Luzzi, known as Mondino (c. 1270–1327), who studied medicine and philosophy and taught at Bologna for a decade from 1314, and who was also a diplomat and politician. Mondino practised systematic dissection and although his knowledge was bounded by Galen he wrote a work of fundamental importance called the *Anathomia*. He explained that the way to begin a dissection was to open up the abdomen by a vertical incision, followed by a horizontal one slightly above the umbilicus; dissections could then be performed, region by region, with careful display of the organs. For three centuries, anatomy lecturers were required by medical schools to use Mondino's text in their teaching.

In Bologna anatomy was taught by surgeons until the sixteenth century when it became an independent study. Mondino's great contributions were that he collected current anatomical ideas into one work, and that he taught anatomy from the human cadaver. But much of his information was sketchy; on the size of the heart, Mondino wrote, 'it is not big and it is not small.'

An Englishman who taught at Montpellier, where the school of medicine began at the end of the tenth century, was Gilbertus Anglicus (1180–1250), who became famous as the author of the *Rosa Anglicana*, which contained extracts from the doctrines of Salernitan and Arab doctors. He suggested as a 'safe' treatment for goitre: 'take a frog when neither the sun nor the moon is shining in the sky; cut off its legs and wrap them in a deerskin; apply the right leg of the frog to the left foot of the patient, and the left leg to the right foot'. But he is remembered for his excellent descriptions of leprosy and smallpox, the contagious nature of which he was one of the first to recognize.

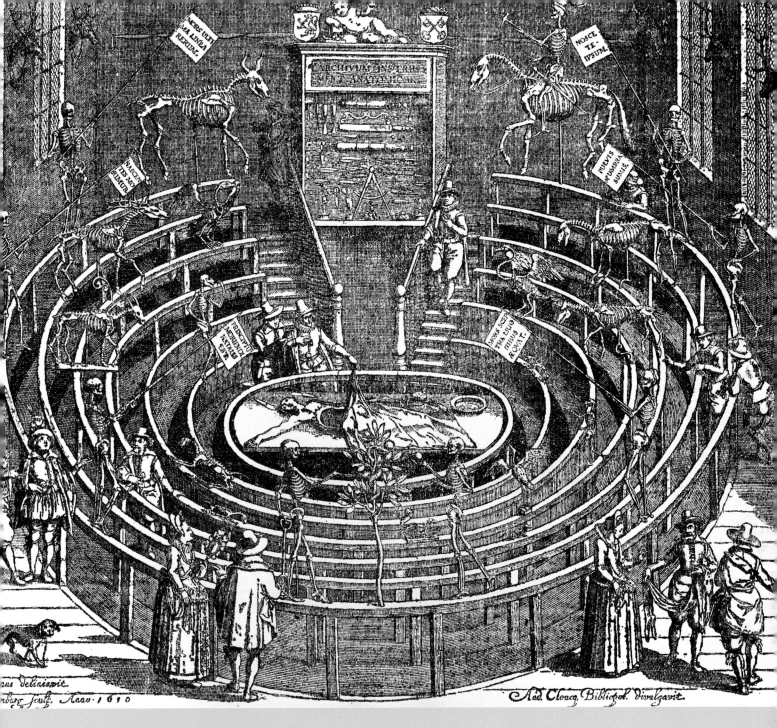

Above: a somewhat fanciful print showing the anatomy theatre at Leiden, in Hollland, in 1610, when it had become a place for the fashionable to visit. The first anatomy theatres were founded towards the end of the sixteenth century.

The greatest and perhaps the most ancient of the universities was at Bologna, where there had been a law school since the eleventh century. It was run on democratic lines, with the students choosing their own professors and electing a rector, who had precedence over everyone, including cardinals, at official functions.

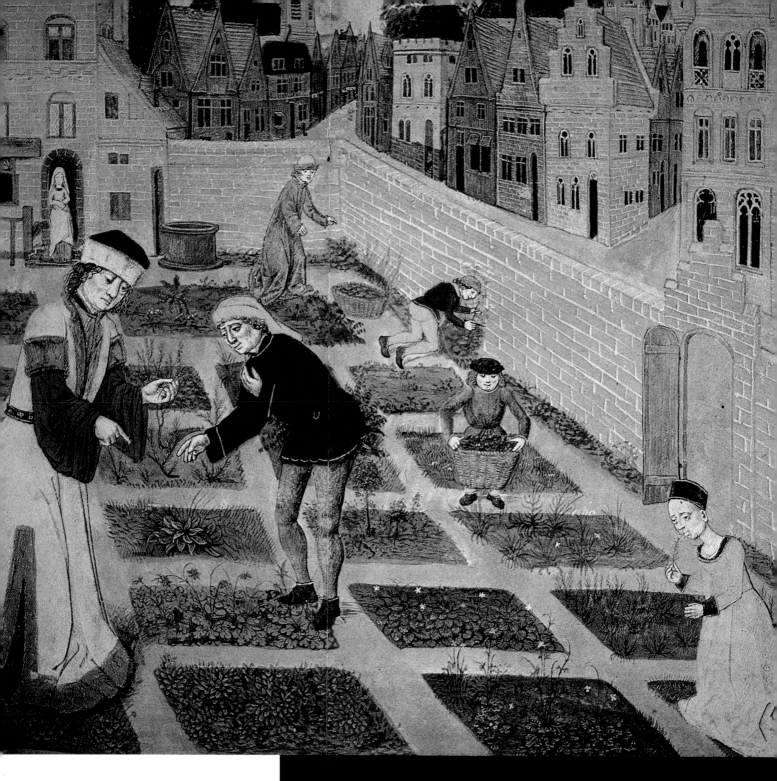

Medical writing of the Middle Ages set great store by astrology. What went on in each part of the body was determined by the influence of the planets and signs of the Zodiac. The sun ruled the right hand side of the body, the moon the left, Venus the neck and abdomen, and so on.

The Paris school of surgery

During the thirteenth century, surgery began to make progress in France. The head of the school of surgery at the university of Paris was the Italian Guido Lanfranc, who was born early in the thirteenth century. Obliged to leave Milan for political reasons, he went to Lyons where he wrote the *Cyrurgia parva* (The little book of surgery). In 1295 he was summoned to Paris to lecture on surgery. He finished writing the *Cyrurgia magna* (The big book of surgery) in 1296 and died early in the fourteenth century.

Lanfranc restored surgery to an honoured place in France. One of the reasons why it was practised largely by itinerant barbers was that physicians thought it beneath their dignity to get blood on their hands. Lanfranc established the principle that no good doctor could ignore surgery and, conversely, that a surgeon was duty bound to acquire some knowledge of medicine. Lanfranc's work was based both on contemporary Italian practice and on his own experience.

The first specifically French work on surgery was by Henri de Mondeville (c.1260–1320) a colleague of Lanfranc's. In the introductory part of his *Chyrurgia*, de Mondeville documented customs of the time in an entertaining manner. He dealt frankly with the question of fees, advising brother surgeons always to ask more than doctors did, and putting them on their guard against rich patients who appeared in old clothes in order to be let off lightly.

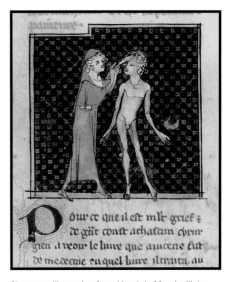

Above: an illustration from Henri de Mondeville's *Chyrurgia*. De Mondeville was court physician to both Philip the Fair and Louis X of France.

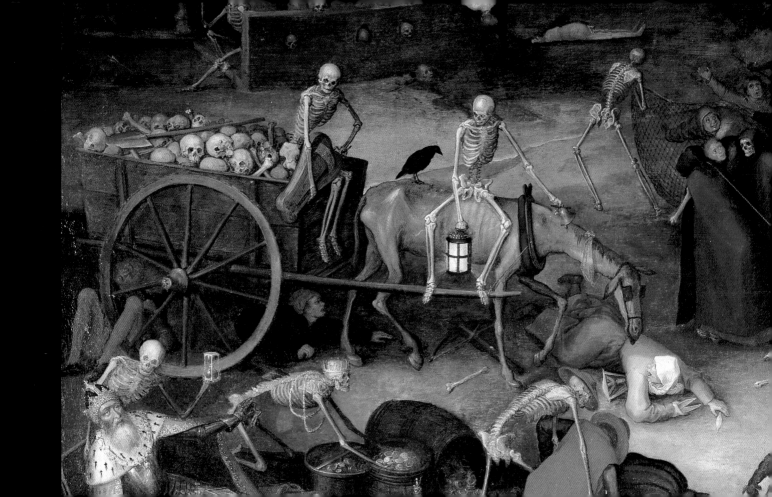

PLAGUES AND PANDEMICS

When the Black Death came to Europe, astrologers rapidly reached agreement over its cause, stating that it was the result of the conjunction of Saturn, Jupiter and Mars. The Franciscan monk Michele di Piazza wrote that the plague was spread '*propter infectionem hanelitus*' (by infection of the breath). This statement is significant in using the term infection for the first time, though in too generic a sense to have a specific implication.

The Christian Era has witnessed three pandemics of plague. The first spread through Europe from the East during the reign of Justinian in 542 and 543; the second, the Black Death, reached England in 1348; while the third, which began in 1894, started in China and on reaching Hong Kong in May 1894 spread rapidly throughout most parts of the world, but in Europe and America deaths were comparatively few.

All these plagues were characterized by enormously high death rates. There is little documentary evidence to give a reliable figure for the casualties of the first, but it has been estimated that a quarter of the population of Europe, or 25,000,000 people, died in the Black Death; in some places the population was reduced by three-quarters in the first pestilence.

Like the first pandemic, the Black Death came from the East. It is thought that the first Europeans to be affected were the Italian merchants who traded in central Asia and fled from the Tartars to Caffa (now Feodosiya) in the Crimea, a Genoese trading port. Caffa was besieged for three years, during which time the plague broke out among the Tartars. Dead bodies were catapulted inside the walls and, after the Tartars had dispersed, the surviving Italians returned home by ship, apparently healthy but in fact carriers of the deadly pestilence which immediately broke out in Genoa.

61...

From Genoa the plague spread throughout Italy; the start of its progress was described by Fra Michele di Piazza, the author of *Historia Sicula ab anno 1337 ad annum 1361* (History of Sicily 1337–1361):

'In the first days of October 1347, the year of the Incarnation of the Son of God, twelve Genoese galleys fleeing before the wrath of our Lord over their wicked deeds, entered the port of Messina. The sailors brought in their bones a disease so violent that whoever spoke a word to them was infected and could in no way save himself from death. Those to whom the disease was transmitted by infection of the breath were stricken with pains all over the body and felt a terrible lassitude. Then there appeared, on a thigh or an arm, a pustule like a lentil. From this the infection penetrated the body and violent bloody vomiting began. It lasted for a period of three days and there was no way of preventing its ending in death.'

The Genoese ships were subsequently expelled from the port but the infection remained, depopulating the town.

Plague reached Florence in 1348. Boccaccio wrote: 'This trouble struck such terrible fear into the hearts of men and women that brothers deserted each other, an uncle left his nephew and a sister left her brother; women often abandoned their husbands and worse, incredible though it is, fathers and mothers acted towards their children as if they were not their own, by refusing to see them or look after them.'

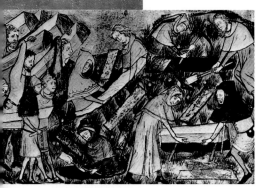

Top: a detail from The Triumph of Death, a copy by Jan Breughel of the painting by his father, Pieter.

Above: burial of the dead in Tournai, Flanders, 1349. Later, in order to keep pace with the huge numbers of the dead, bodies were frequently buried in communal graves. Coffins became a luxury, bodies were often naked or at best wrapped in coarse shrouds.

Far left: a woodcut showing a doctor lancing a bubo. Abcesses and carbuncles, particularly in the groin and armpits, were symptoms of the Black Death.

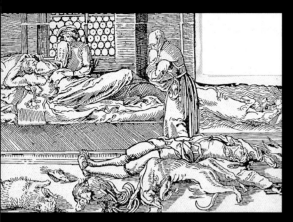

Above: plague, an illusttration by Hans Weiditz from *The Remedies of Petrach*, 1520. A dying patient is comforted while a doctor looks on. The dead, both men and animals, lie on the floor.

Below: The Flagellants of Doornik, Netherlands, a coloured miniature dated 1349.

... 6 2

The first English town to be affected by the plague, in August 1348, was Weymouth, and from here the Black Death soon spread to Bristol. Spread eastwards occurred rapidly, and London was attacked in November. East Anglia and the north were affected in the following spring and summer. By the end of 1349 the Black Death was over, but it had had the devastating effects of reducing the English population by perhaps a third, and of establishing epidemic plague, which persisted for a period of three hundred years.

We know, from many contemporary accounts, of the gravely demoralizing effect of this terrible pestilence on superstitious people ignorant of its nature, which led to strange psychic epidemics as well as physical ones. Thus, among other grotesque developments, there arose the confraternity of the Flagellants. In long cloaks, with a scarlet cross on their breasts, these fanatics passed in procession through the town and countryside, flogging themselves with three-tailed lashes in the belief that the Lord would be moved to compassion by their suffering and would end the plague. Wherever they went, the Flagellants made converts and these frenetic bands themselves became a plague, committing vandalism, looting, arson and rape. On reaching Avignon, they were threatened with excommunication by Pope Clement V.

Preventive measures in the years when the plague was devastating Europe were on a very small scale, as might be expected with people so resigned to their fate. In some towns the authorities attempted to isolate the plague-stricken away from any dwellings, and to isolate for ten days anyone who had treated those infected by the contagion. Milan and Venice refused access to any suspect persons or goods. Doctors, for their own protection, had adopted a mode of dress that made them look rather like great birds of prey; the effect was heightened by a beak-like facepiece that was in reality a sponge soaked in vinegar and aromatic substances held in front of the nose.

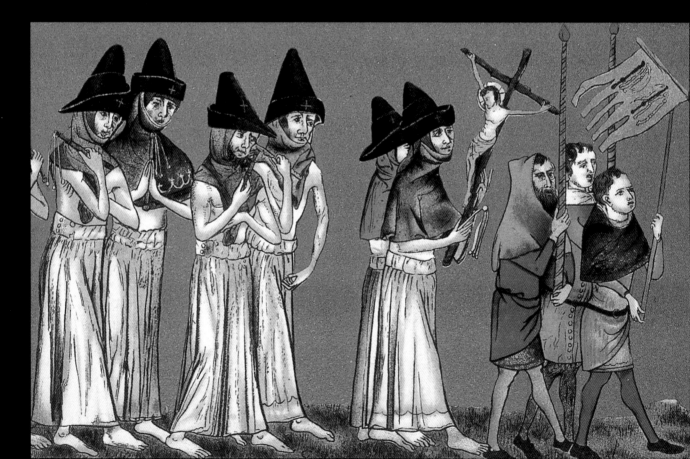

Besides the Black Death, dancing mania, St Vitus' dance, St Anthony's fire (ergotism), *sudor Anglicus* (the English sweating sickness) and scrofula (king's evil) were among the plagues that devasted Europe.

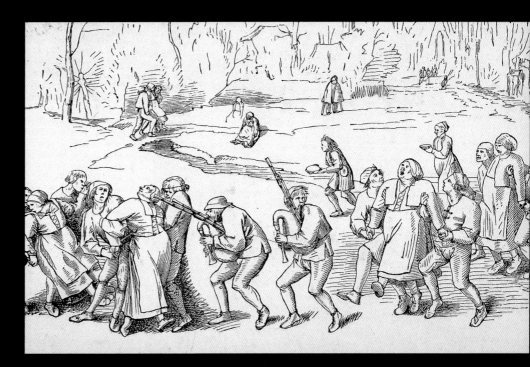

Above: a drawing by Pieter Brueghel, 1564, showing victims of St Vitus' dance making their way in pilgrimage to Echternach, in Luxembourg.

63...

'Leprosy' and other epidemics

As the imagined aides of the devil, who was assumed to be the cause of the plague, Jews and lepers became scapegoats. Thus in many parts of Europe, but especially Switzerland and Alsace, Jews were massacred together with those lepers who had escaped the plague.

Just as the word plague was used as a generic term for any epidemic, so in the Middle Ages leprosy was the name given to many skin diseases, doubtless including non-infectious conditions such as eczema and psoriasis, as well as diseases like smallpox. It is very likely that few of the green-gowned 'lepers' of mediaeval England, who were excluded from public places and made to wear wooden clappers on the ends of their sleeves to warn of their approach, were suffering from the ravages of *Mycobacterium leprae* (the tuberculosis-like organism discovered by Hansen in 1871). Leprosy is in fact contagious, but is spread only with difficulty. It seems that in Britain true leprosy died out completely by the fifteenth century. Certainly some of the accounts of 'venereal leprosy' in the reign of Edward III sound like secondary syphilis.

After the Black Death a new epidemic broke out in Germany; this was the dancing mania. It spread hysterically, at first to people in places where there were victims of St Vitus' dance. It raged through the Low Countries and northern France; the priesthood tried exorcism, convinced it was caused by collective possession by devils.

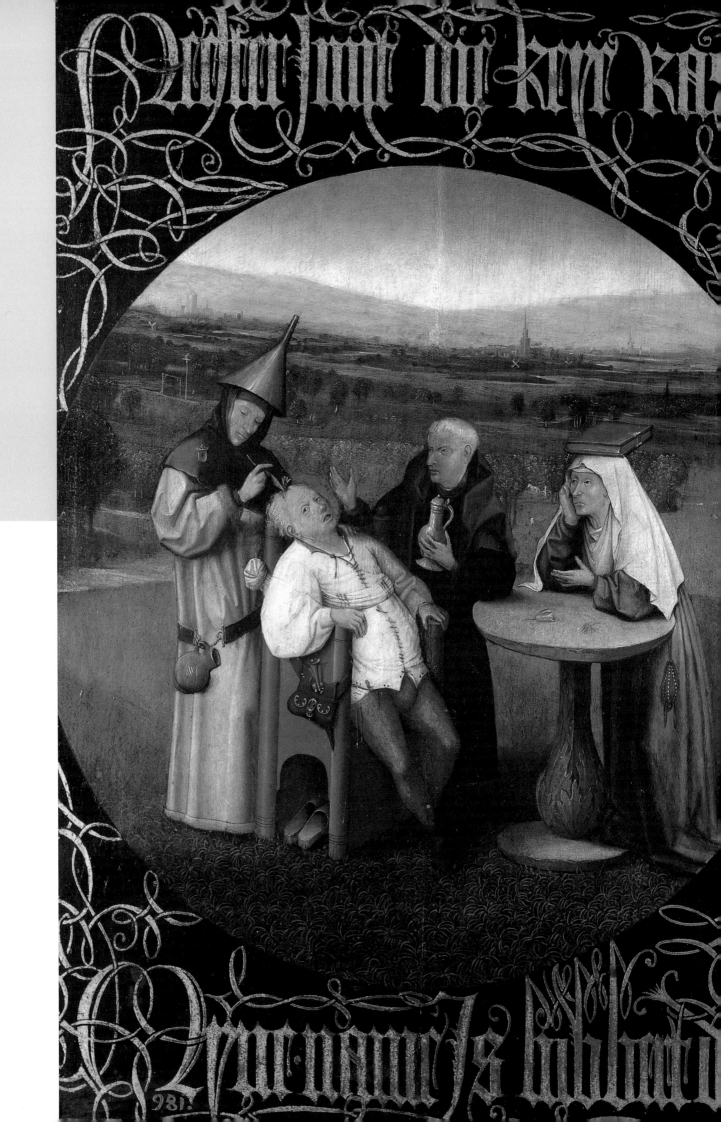

Another epidemic disease which was widespread and much feared during the Middle Ages was the holy fire or St Anthony's fire (ergotism). This manifested itself as progressive gangrene of the limbs and ended in loss of limbs and death. It was first mentioned in the middle of the ninth century, and there were at least six outbreaks up to 1129. It was then realized that the epidemic broke out in years when rye ripened badly; the condition has almost disappeared now, thanks to advances in the processing of flour and the discovery of the causative agent *Claviceps purpurea*, a fungus which infects the grain and produces a toxic substance.

Towards the middle of the fifeeenth century, a serious epidemic disease broke out in England; this was *sudor Anglicus* or the English sweating sickness. The first outbreak took place among the victorious forces of Henry VII after Bosworth Field in 1485 and it spread rapidly all over England, affecting the young and fit, and the devastation was so great that, as Holinshed wrote, 'scarce one amongst an hundred that sickened did escape with life; for all in manner as soone as the sweat took them or in a short time after yielding up the ghost'. It recurred in 1507 and 1517, and spread to Calais, and most virulently of all, in 1529, when Europe as far as Vienna was devastated. The last outbreak took place in 1551 and was confined to England.

John Caius, president of the Royal College of Physicians in London, wrote an account of the sickness in 1552, which was in fact the first English monograph on any disease. The disease remains unidentified, it has been suggested that it may have been a form of typhus.

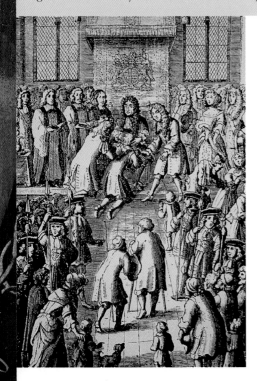

Far left: Removal of the Stone of Folly by Hieronymus Bosch. Stone-cutters were itinerants who claimed to cure all mental disorders by removing stones from the head of the sufferer. They would make a slight incision in the scalp and then 'remove' the stone and noisily throw it into a bucket.

Left: Charles II, one of the last English kings to practise the art of touching patients suffering from scrofula or king's evil.

65...

Medicine and suggestion

As is plain, the Middle Ages were exceptionally troubled times. Medicine had little help to offer. Pathology was still based on the doctrine of the humours, and so diagnosis rested on examination of the blood, urine and sputum. Consequently treatment consisted of blood-letting, purging, emetics, enemas and blistering – all debilitating procedures liable to turn the scales against the sick patient. Magic and suggestion were major therapeutic tools, and, at a time when impotence, loss of memory, hysteria and other complaints were attributable to possession by the devil or to witchcraft, it was natural that exorcism should come within the sphere of therapeutic practice.

Scrofula, tuberculous enlargement of lymph glands in the neck, was known as king's evil and was treated in England and France by the king's touch. According to English sources, the first king to cure this condition was Edward the Confessor (1002–66), but the French say it was Clovis in the year 496, when he was crowned king of the Franks. The practice continued until the eighteenth century. William of Orange is said to have touched only one victim, saying 'may God give you better health and more sense'.

GUILDS, PHARMACIES AND HOSPITALS

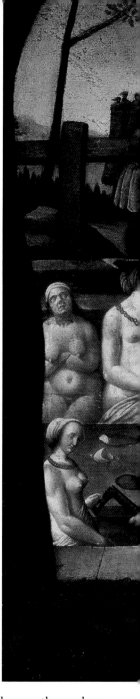

In the late Middle Ages, medicine, which was still developing along the lines of the school of Salerno, passed entirely into the hands of the laity: Pope Honorius III had in fact forbidden the clergy to practise. The physicians started to organize themselves into professional bodies, with rights protected by the law of the land, for this was the period of the formation of the guilds, which exercised strict regulations over the trades and professions.

The status of physicians in society improved, but, in practice, little had changed. Pathology was still based on the theory of humours, while diagnosis, except in a few rare cases, was usually based on interpretation of the colour, density and smell of the blood, of the smell and colour of the sputum, and above all on examination of the urine. There were innumerable systems, each explaining how detailed diagnosis of all types of diseases could be determined not only from the colour and odour of the urine, but from the layers of sediment formed in the collecting flask. The diagnosis was often optimistically simple: cloudiness in the upper layer indicated that the seat of the disease was in the head, in the lower layer conditions of the bladder or genital organs.

Therapy was still based on the theory of opposites (*contraria contrariis*), as it had been in Galen's day, so that for diseases thought to be caused by excess of bodily fluid (plethora), blood-letting was the main treatment. This procedure was supposed to deflect the material causing the illness and make it pass from one organ to another. When blood was taken from the side of the body opposite that where the disease was situated it was revulsive, but when taken from the same side as the disease, derivative, tending to relieve the patient's plethora and pain. The most detailed directions were given regarding the most favourable days and hours for blood-letting, the correct veins to be tapped, also the amount of blood to be taken and the number of bleedings. Blood was usually taken by opening a vein with a lancet, but sometimes by blood-sucking leeches or with the use of cupping vessels.

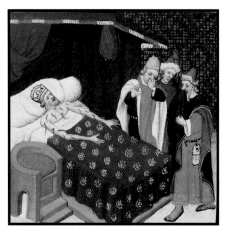

Above: blood-letting with leeches, from a manuscript of Bocaccio's *Decameron*. Special diets were prescribed for use before and after blood-letting.

Blood-letting was often performed at public baths, which were themselves a popular form of therapy. Some baths were enormous tanks in which the bathers stood or sat, others were steam baths, in which the patients were covered to the neck with a cloth while steam was introduced from below. Bathing was often mixed, and was often made the occasion for feasting and drinking, so that in time it became associated with debauchery. In the early sixteenth century, increasing knowledge of the nature of contagion led to regulations suppressing mixed bathing, and the use of communal baths gradually died out.

Barbers, who performed many of the functions of the doctor, including blood-letting, purging and tooth-drawing, were important figures in medicine right up to the seventeenth and even eighteenth century. By the end of the Middle Ages the barber-surgeons were well established, and in 1505 the faculty of medicine in Paris instituted a course for barbers, to spite the surgeons proper, of whom it was jealous; in the course of time the barbers became more closely associated with the physicians. In England, in 1462, the large and prosperous Guild of Barbers became the Company of Barbers, while the surgeons obtained a special charter in 1492. Under Henry VIII, in 1540, the Barber Company was joined with the small and exclusive Guild of Surgeons to become the United Barber-Surgeon Company.

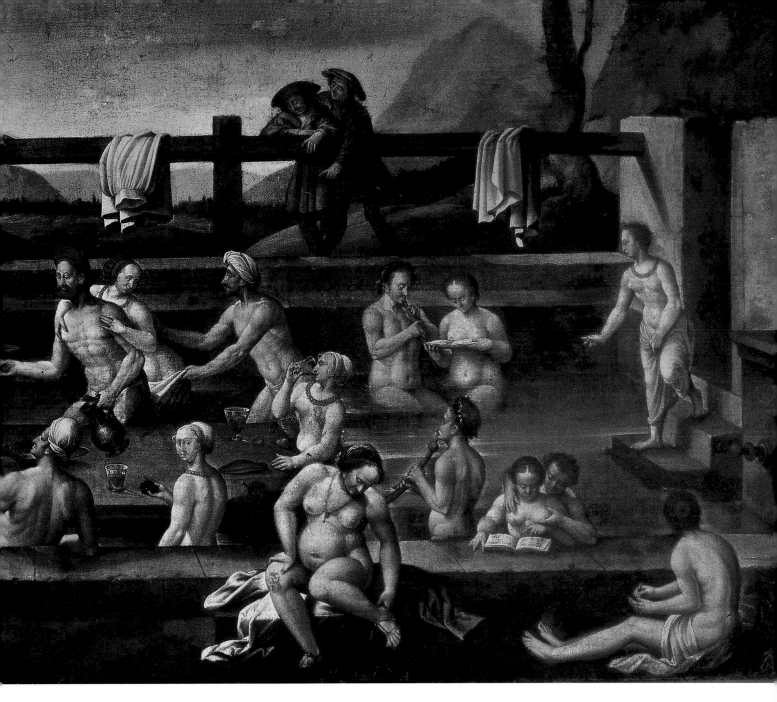

Above: the baths at Leuk, in Switzerland, by Hans Boch the Elder. Mixed bathing was especially popular in the Germanic countries.

Blood-letting was often performed at public baths, which were themselves a popular form of therapy. Bathing was often mixed, and frequently the occasion for feasting and drinking, so it became associated with debauchery. As knowledge of the nature of contagion increased, the use of communal baths gradually died out.

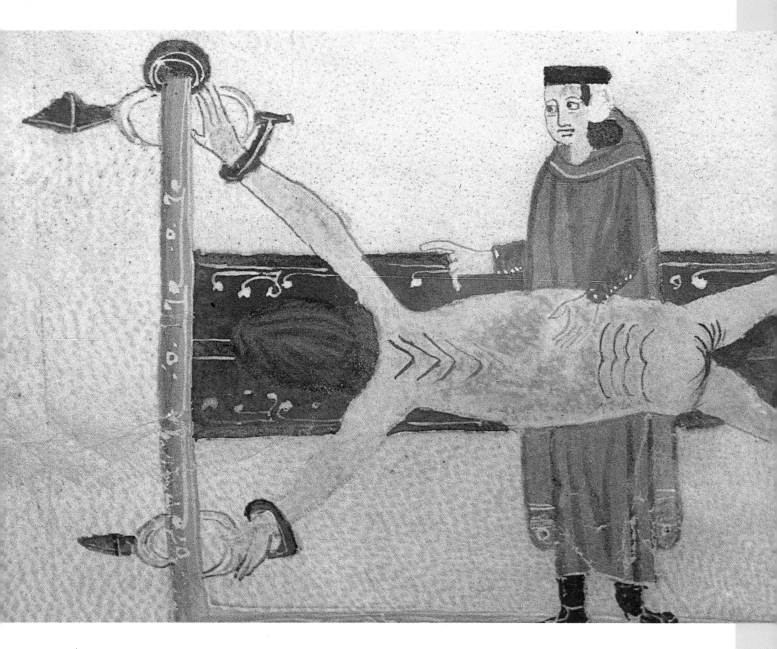

Above: a thirteenth-century surgeon stands by an operating table. Barbers, who doubled as surgeons, had probably begun to gain their importance around 1100, when monks went regularly to the barbers for their tonsure and also for bleeding, which church law required them to undergo regularly.

The drugs used in treatment came from many sources, including plants. At the same time, there was widespread use of various complicated prescriptions containing innumerable constituents from precious stones to viper's flesh. The most famous was 'theriacrum', said to have been invented by Nero's physician, which contained fifty-seven ingredients.

Italy, towards the end of the thirteenth century, saw the establishment of the first public pharmacies. Based on the Arab model, they developed originally in the monasteries and courts, later to become private shops where physicians came not only to buy drugs but also to meet colleagues and even to see patients. The pharmacist himself was often an astrologer or alchemist who became the centre of a sort of scientific circle.

The drugs used in treatment were drawn from all sources, especially from plants, and many preparations with genuine pharmacological properties were known. At the same time, there was widespread use of various complicated prescriptions containing innumerable constituents from precious stones to vipers' flesh, which had to be compounded according to the most rigid and nonsensical instructions; the most fashionable was 'theriacum', said to have been invented by Nero's physician, which contained fifty-seven substances. Many of the drugs were imported from the Orient, and as they formed light and compact cargoes they became one of the most important factors in the growth of trade and the opening up of new sea routes.

Hospitals can be traced back in one form or another as far as ancient Greece, but the institution as we know it today was probably a product of the Christian principle of charity. The Middle Ages saw the founding of hundreds of hospitals all over Europe and in the lands visited by the Crusades. One of the most important developments was the widespread foundation of leper hospitals; at the height of the epidemic era there were over two hundred in England and Scotland and about two thousand in France.

About the beginning of the thirteenth century, the hospitals began to pass from the hands of the church to the civic authorities. This was the period which saw the expansion of the great city hospitals, like the Hôtel-Dieu in Paris, the Santo Spirito in Rome and St Bartholomew's and St Thomas's in London. Cities lavished great wealth on these buildings, particularly in Italy, where many of the great architects and artists of the day were commissioned to design them. This inspired patronage formed the foundations of an association between medicine and the arts which was to bear such rich fruit in the glorious age of the Renaissance.

69...

Right: the four virtues, Temperance, Prudence, Fortitude and Justice, instructing the nuns at the Hôtel-Dieu in the art of nursing. An illustration from a mediaeval manuscript.

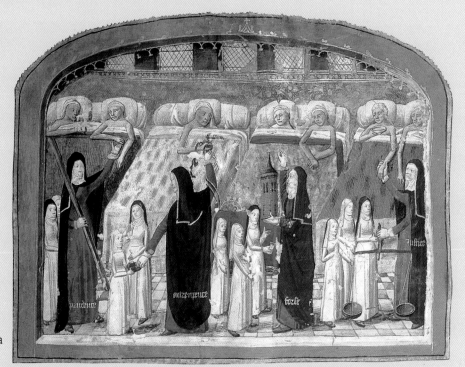

MEDICINE AND HUMANISM

With the end of the Middle Ages, a cultural movement began characterized by the revival of ancient learning through direct study of the work of Greek and Roman authors. This was the beginning of Humanism, within the wider framework of what is known as the Renaissance.

The movement originated in Italy. Interest in classical antiquity was cultivated, while metaphysical speculations ceased and the fetters on learning imposed by the mediaeval attitude to religion fell away. There were repercussions in all aspects of life; in politics, the arts and in science, which flourished as a result of of direct observation of nature, as well as in medicine. Many simultaneous events contributed to this revival of learning. The finite world of the Middle Ages disappeared for ever with the great voyages of Columbus, da Gama and Magellan, and with Copernicus placing the sun at the centre of the universe. Ancient Greek culture and the open-minded rationality of Plato and Hippocrates came to Italy with the scholars fleeing from Constantinople after its fall to the Turks in 1453, but perhaps the most powerful single factor was the invention of printing and its rapid spread through Europe.

The great physicians of the period were humanists and men of letters. Although astrology was used, and diagnosis and treatment depended on examination of the urine and on blood-letting, and quacks of every description still flourished, nevertheless the best doctors were held in high esteem.

Doctors came from the wealthier classes. They were educated at the universities, and those of Italy were now at their zenith and students flocked from abroad. Initially, many teachers expressed conservative views, and Galen and Avicenna were still the standard authors. Nevertheless, new attitudes began to make themselves evident. Dissection was practised more and more, and although the old custom persisted of reading from the pages of Galen while a dissector displayed the organs, ignoring the discrepancies between text and fact, the anatomical knowledge made available to students gradually increased. More and more teachers carried out dissections themselves, but until the end of the century anatomy was always taught together with surgery, and it was only in 1570 that the first separate chairs for the two subjects were created.

Anatomy was to be revitalised in the sixteenth century with the work of Leonardo and Vesalius, but from the time of Mondino many crude attempts at depicting the organs of the body had appeared in print. None of the illustrations in books printed before 1539 represented original observations or research, but were mostly copies of old manuscript drawings. In the Middle Ages anatomy was usually shown in five schematic pictures, illustrating the skeleton and nervous, muscular, arterial and venous systems. Such mediaeval drawings were diagrammatic memory aids, and contained medical folk-lore as well as fanciful ideas. Zodiacal pictures representing diseases and wounds were produced unchanged over hundreds of years. In contrast to these crude and inaccurate drawings produced for doctors, the portrayal of human anatomy by the great Florentine painters of the fifteenth century reached a state of perfection. Perspective, geometry and human proportions were studied assiduously, and an interest in dissection grew since the artists formed part of the Florentine Guild of Physicians and Apothecaries, bringing painters, apothecaries and physicians into close contact.

The Middle Ages disappeared for ever with the great voyages of da Gama, Columbus and Magellan, and with Copernicus placing the sun at the centre of the universe.

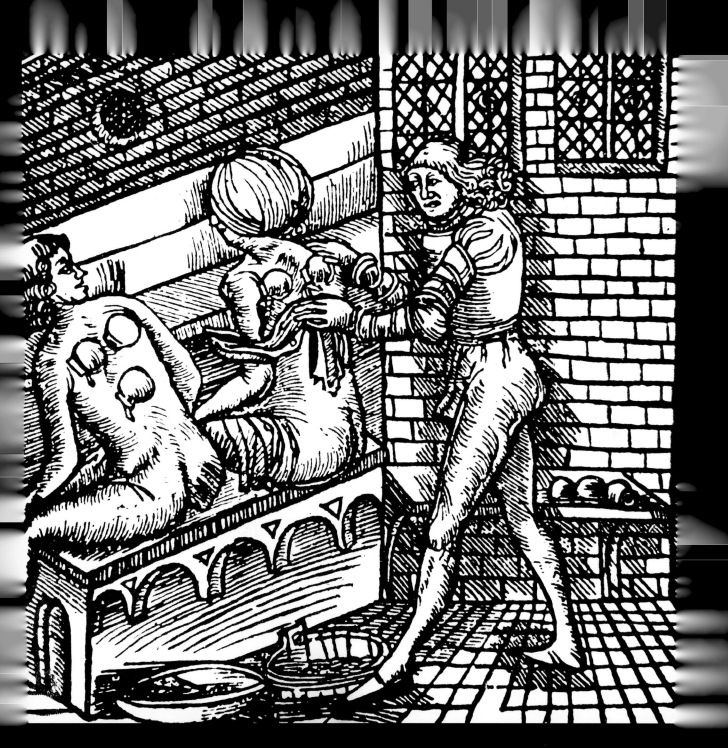

Above: cupping was a treatment which dated back to the Romans. Wet cupping involved making superficial incisions in the skin, a small piece of lint was then placed in a metal or glass cup and the cup applied to the skin. The burning created a vacuum and blood could be drawn. This process was also known as the artificial leech. In dry cupping, the skin was not cut, but the suction was regarded as sufficient to extract the vicious humour.

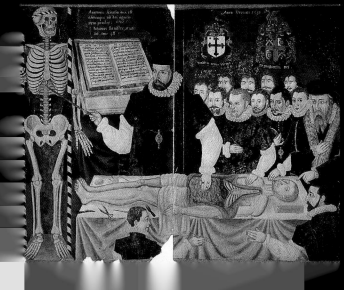

Left: Dr John Bannister, an Elizabethan scholar, delivering an anatomy lecture. A painting dated 1581.

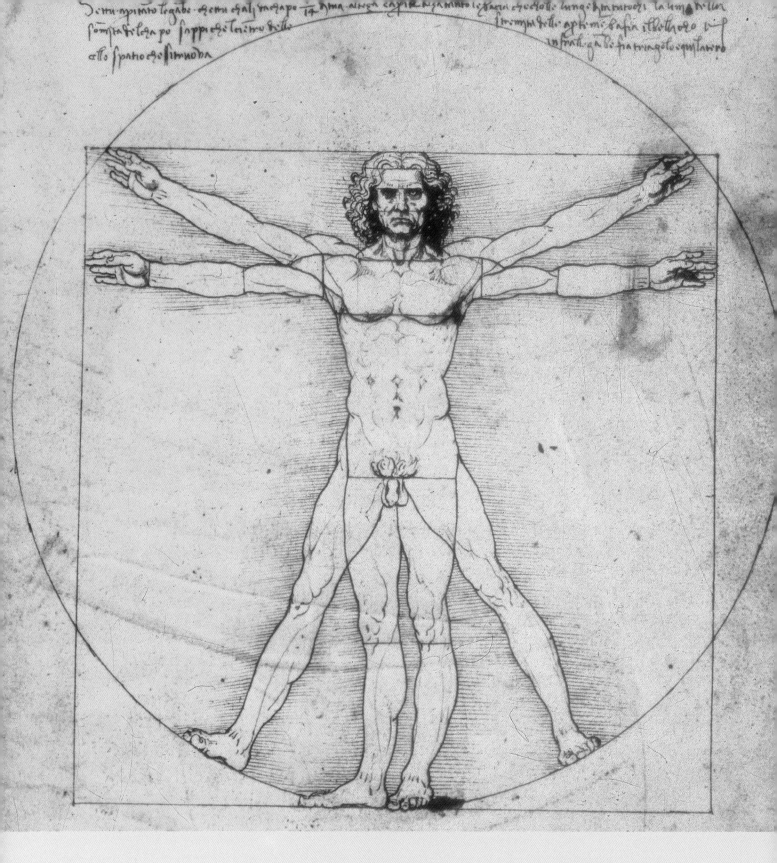

Leonardo's drawings show him to be
the creator both of medical illustration
and of art in relation to physiology.
His powers of observation and stupendous
technical skill make him, historically
speaking, the father of anatomy.

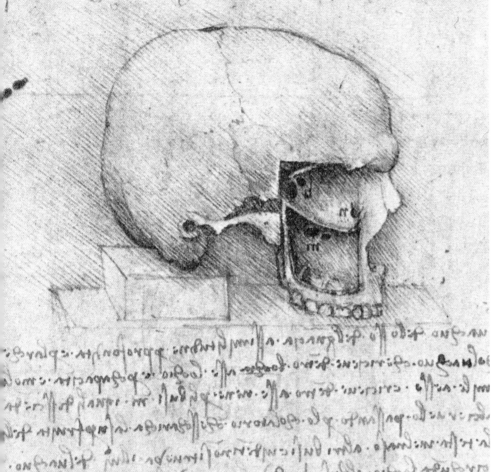

ART AND ANATOMY

Leonardo da Vinci, who excelled in both the arts and the sciences, approached anatomy without preconceptions, relying solely on his own observation and experiment. When he was in the service of the Borgia family in Rome, he dissected more than thirty bodies by candlelight in the mortuary of the Santo Spirito, producing a thousand drawings of his dissections. One anatomical technique he devised is still employed; that of injecting liquid wax into the body cavities to reveal their exact structure. In this way, he studied the heart, lungs and womb, and became the first person to attempt to trace the course of the cranial nerves and to dissect the foetal membranes.

Above left: the proportions of the human figure, the so-called 'Vitruvian man' by Leonardo.

Above right: the human skull. A drawing from the huge collection of Leonardo's drawings in the collection of H M the Queen at Windsor Castle.

Leonardo analysed the muscular system and recognized the specific action of each muscle, and studied the valves of the veins. He also made drawings of the coronary arteries and their course, but did not grasp correctly the place of the septum dividing the right and left parts of the heart; had he done so he might have discovered the circulation of the blood.

Leonardo da Vinci was recognized in his lifetime as a genius for his paintings and drawings, and also as an architect, engineer, scientist and inventor. He might also have been regarded as the father of anatomy, had his notebooks not lain undiscovered for two centuries. From the drawings and notes in them it seems that he intended to write a major treatise on anatomy, in collaboration with Marc Antonio della Torre of Verona, to whom Vasari attributed the attempt to break new ground in the teachings of anatomy.

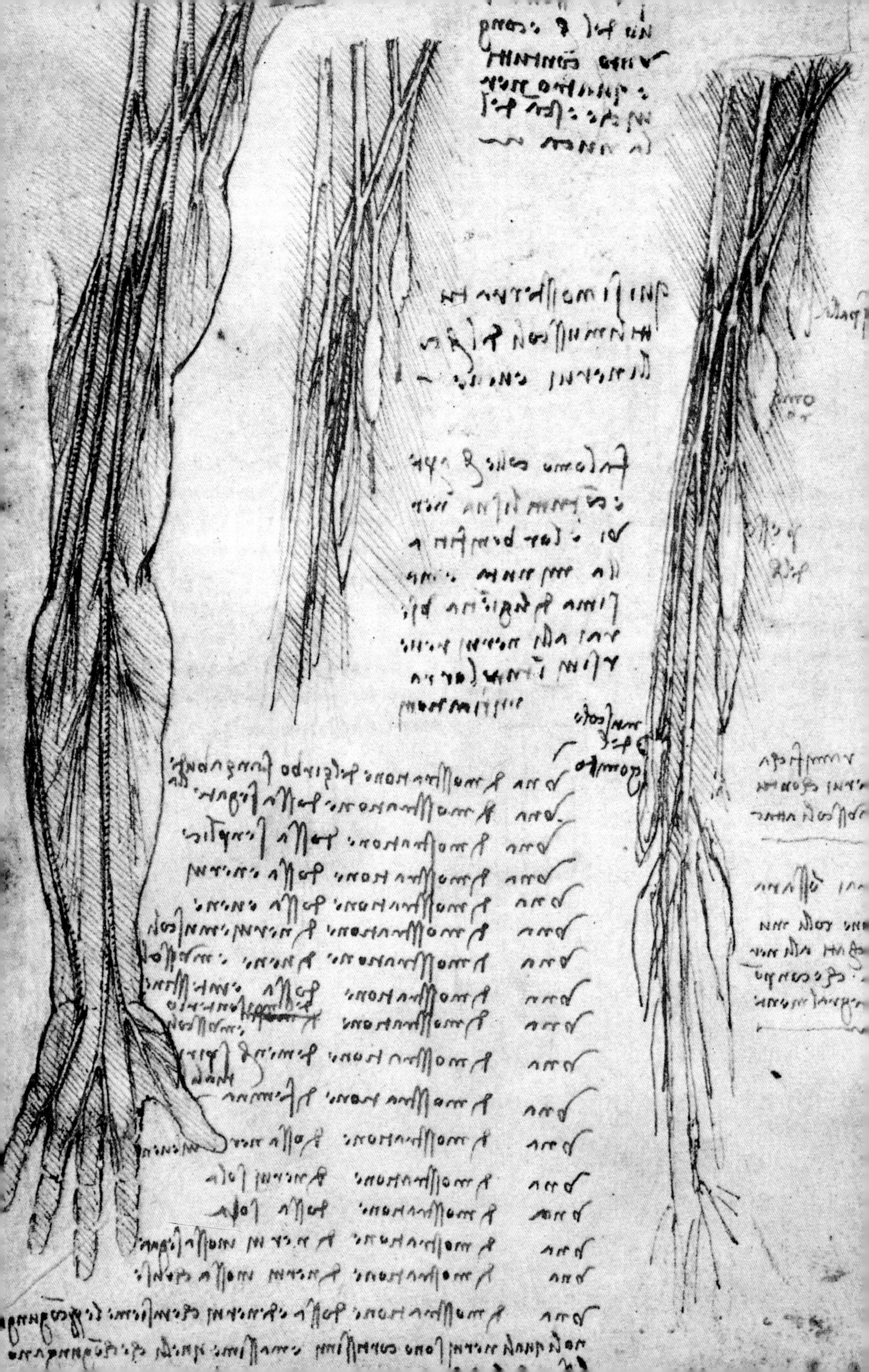

'I have dissected more than ten human bodies, destroying all the various members and removing the minutest particles of flesh which surrounded these veins, without causing any effusion of blood other than the imperceptible bleeding of the capilliary veins.'

These drawings show Leonardo to be the creator both of medical illustration and also of anatomy in relation to physiology, and his scientific objectivity combined with his superb powers of independent observation and stupendous technical skill make him, historically speaking, the father of anatomy. Passages from his notebooks contain his justification of anatomical illustration and, by stressing the need for presenting collected facts in an easily comprehensible and unequivocal form, he shows himself to be a true scientist.

75...

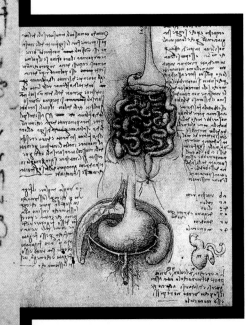

Above left: three studies of the arm, and, above: a study of the digestive system and a study of the stomach, liver and spleen; two more of Leonardo's anatomical drawings from the magnificent collection of H M the Queen at Windsor Castle.

'You who say that it is better to watch an anatomical demonstration than to see these drawings, you would be right if it were possible to observe all the details shown in such drawings in a single figure, in which with all your cleverness you will not see or acquire knowledge of more than some few veins, while in order to obtain a true and complete knowledge of these, I have dissected more than ten human bodies, destroying all the various members and removing the minutest particles of flesh which surrounded these veins, without causing any effusion of blood other than the imperceptible bleeding of the capillary veins. And as one single body did not suffice for so long a time, it was necessary to proceed by stages with so many bodies as would render my knowledge complete; this I repeated twice in order to discover the differences. And though you should have love for such things you may perhaps be deterred by natural repugnance, and if this does not prevent you, you may perhaps be deterred by fear of passing the night hours in the company of these corpses, quartered and flayed and horrible to behold; and if this does not deter you, then perhaps you may lack the skill in drawing, essential for such representation; and if you had the skill in drawing, it may not be combined with a knowledge of perspective; and if it is so combined you may not understand the methods of geometrical demonstration and the methods of estimating the force and strength of muscles; or perhaps you may be wanting in patience so that you will not be diligent.'

The study of anatomy, and with it medical knowledge, was at last on the right road. Not only medical students, but every great artist learned anatomy and some became skilled anatomists.

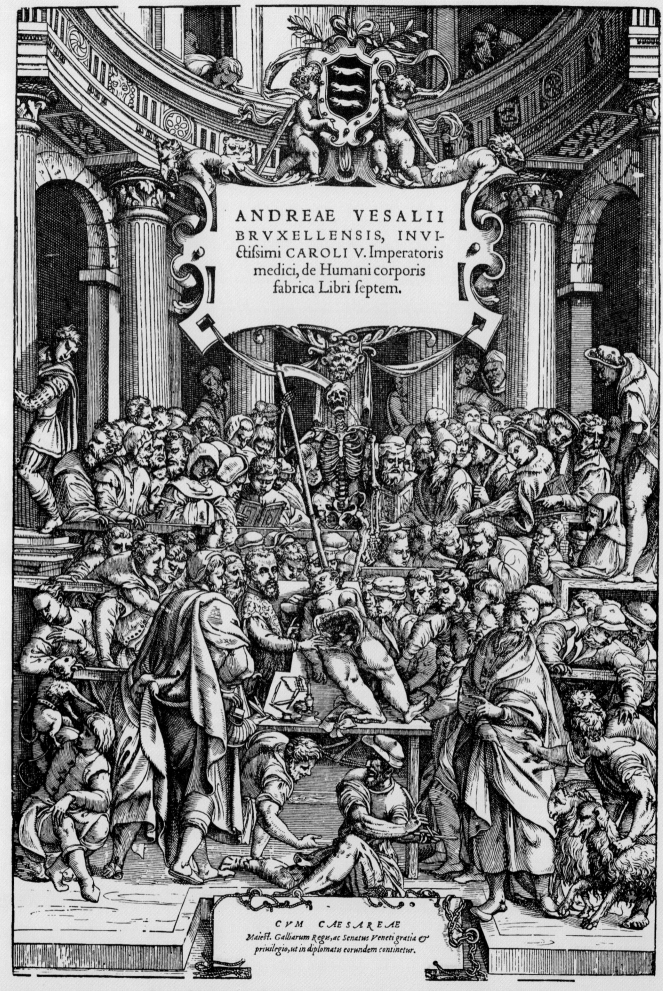

ANDREAE VESALII
BRVXELLENSIS, INVI-
ctifsimi CAROLI V. Imperatoris
medici, de Humani corporis
fabrica Libri septem.

CVM CAESAREAE
Maieft. Galliarum Regis, ac Senatus Veneti gratia &
priuilegio, ut in diplomatis eorundem continetur.

BASILEAE, PER IOANNEM OPORINVM.

VESALIUS AND THE END OF GALENISM

The man who is celebrated as the father of anatomy was not Leonardo da Vinci, but a Fleming called Andreas Vesalius (1514–63), the son of an apothecary. He studied at Louvain, Montpellier and Paris, and in 1537 he went to Padua to join a compatriot, Stephen Calcar, who was studying painting under Titian. Calcar made superb illustrations for Vesalius's works, thereby contributing a good deal to the fame of the anatomist himself. The same year, Vesalius was appointed to the chair of medicine and anatomy at Padua and in 1538 his work *Tabulae anatomicae sex* (Six anatomical tables) was published with both text and illustrations containing the age-old errors of Galen.

Over the next five years, Vesalius discarded the dogma of Galen and in 1543, when he was just twenty-eight, he finished his monumental work, *De humani corporis fabrica libri septem* (Seven books on the structure of the human body), which was printed at Basle. It caused an unprecedented uproar; most of the teachers at the university were Galenists and they sided against him, violently denying the truth of Vesalius's work.

When he was a mere twenty-eight, Vesalius published his monumental work, *De humani corporis,* the foundation of modern medicine.

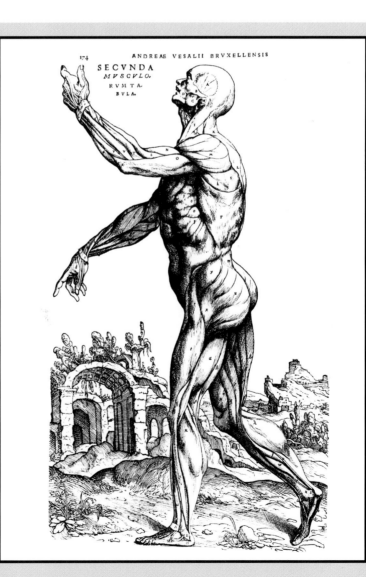

77...

Left: the title page of *De humani corporis,* showing Vesalius in a lofty anatomy theatre dissecting a female patient. Vesalius was closely involved with the production of the book, choosing the paper and supervising the engravings.

Right: the muscular structure of man, a plate from *De humani corporis.*

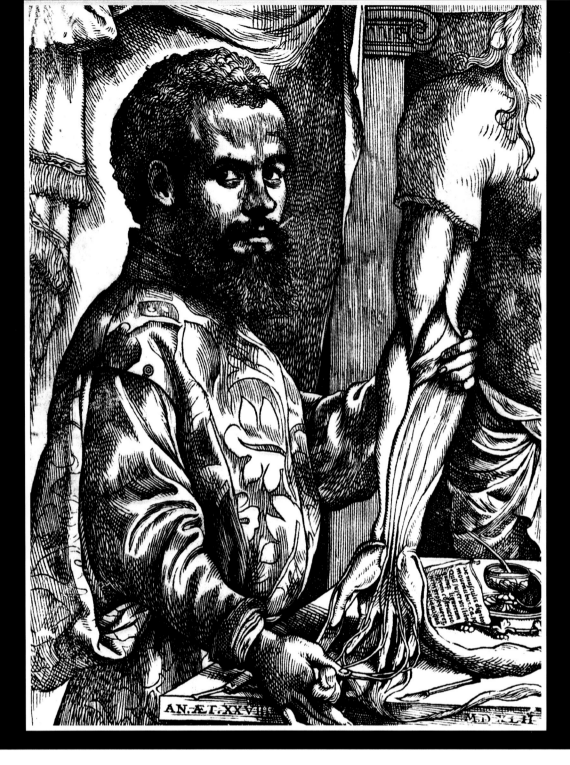

Vesalius showed where previous teachers had erred, but he had no wish to triumph for personal reasons. The sea of ignorance facing him was vast, and he also had the ill-will of his accusers to contend with. Unable to withstand them, irritated by his colleagues and threatened by the Church, he gathered together all his unpublished work and burned it. He then left Padua to become physician to the Emperor Charles V, and later to Philip II of Spain. A brilliant scientific career was over.

Some little time passed before other scholars began to appreciate Vesalius's work at its true worth. The revelation of Galen's fundamental errors was a tremendous shock. The worst of the errors was related to the anatomy of the liver, bile duct, upper jaw and uterus. What upset the Galenists most of all was Vesalius's denial of the existence of the pores in the septum through which blood was supposed to flow from the right to the left ventricle of the heart. It is strange that Galen, who after all made numerous dissections, should have erred also in the description of such parts of the skeleton as the sternum, sacrum and articular cartilages of the knee. Naturally, Vesalius's work itself was not entirely free of errors. He had not fathomed the mechanism of circulation; he placed the lens in the centre of the eyeball; he believed the vena cava came from the liver; that there was a muscle inside the nose and seven (not twelve) cranial nerves. However, these and other faults did not stop the new work done by this great anatomist from producing positive long-term results, and *De humani corporis* must be regarded as one of the most important books ever published, and the foundation of modern medicine.

Although he was a superb observer and undoubtedly a man of great learning, as an innovator Vesalius was not so very far ahead of some of his colleagues, such as Jacopo Berengario da Carpi (1470–1550), the son of a famous surgeon and a pupil of Aldus Manutius, founder of the Aldine Press in Venice. Berengario studied at Bologna, taught at Pavia and Bologna, and practised in Rome and in Ferrara. His heirs inherited his considerable wealth, obtained largely from treatment of patients with syphilis; he was among the first to popularize the use of mercurial ointments in the treatment of this disease.

Although thoroughly unscrupulous, according to Benvenuto Cellini who knew him well, Berengario was a very accurate anatomist. In 1518 he published *De fractura calvariae sive cranii* (On fracture of the cranium), which was followed in 1521 by *Commentaria super anatomia Mundini* (Commentary on the anatomy of Mondino), a broadly based and most original work. The *Isagogae*, an anatomical compendium, appeared in 1522 and featured some magnificent illustrations of the heart.

Above: the skeleton, from *De humani corporis*. Despite the liberal intellectual climate of the Renaissance, the study of the human body brought problems. Almost all the anatomists, including Vesalius, were accused of performing dissections on living people.

Left: a wood-cut portrait of Vesalius by Stephen Calcar from the first edition of *De humani corporis*. Calcar, Vesalius's fellow Fleming, was a superb illustrator and very knowledgeable anatomist, whose skills contributed enormously to the book.

According to the French medical historian Daremberg, the finest original work in anatomy was done not by Vesalius but by Gabriele Fallopio (1523–62) who belonged to the Ferrara school, taught at Pisa, and later became professor of anatomy at Padua.

Gabriele Fallopio was estimable as a scholar and as a person. He spoke of Berengario as 'without doubt the restorer of the art of anatomy, which Vesalius then perfected'. Of the *De humani corporis*, he said that it was Vesalius's divine monument and would last for ever. Then, having praised it, he began correcting the errors in the work; he described the ear and cerebral arteries, which Vesalius confused with the sinuses, and the clitoris and the (Fallopian) tubes that still bear his name. He was the first to describe the circular folds of the small intestine, the inguinal ligament, the chorda tympani, the semicircular canals and the lacrimal duct. In addition he wrote an excellent account of the eye muscles and of the cerebral nerves, and because of his contribution to the study of tissues he has been regarded as the precursor of Malpighi and Bichat. Fallopio's most important book was the *Observationes anatomicae*, first published in Venice in 1561; his *Opera omnia* appeared there in 1584, over twenty years after his death. He died in 1562 at the early age of thirty-nine.

Fallopio studied and taught at the universities of Ferrara, Pisa and finally at Padua, where he was succeeded by his pupil Gerolamo Fabrizio d'Acquapendente (c.1533–1619), called Fabricius. Famous in his day as a surgeon, Fabricius was also a great anatomist and physiologist. He was the first to give a good description of the valves of the veins, although he thought that the blood in the veins flowed away from the heart. His best work was done on reproduction, childbirth and the anatomy and physiology of the foetus.

SYPHILIS AND EARLY THEORIES OF INFECTION

In the last years of the fifteenth century, a terrible new epidemic appeared, a lethal infection which produced hideous rashes and ulcers and was spread by sexual contact. It became rife when the army of Charles VIII of France invaded Italy, and was first known as the Neapolitan disease, for a major outbreak occurred among the troops when Naples surrendered and surviving mercenaries returned home, bringing the name and the disease with them. Morbus Gallicus became the term in general use until Girolamo Fracastoro (1478–1553) published in 1530 his poem entitled *Syphilis sive morbus gallicus* (Syphilis or the French disease), in which a young shepherd, Syphilis, insults Apollo; in revenge the god causes the flesh to fall from the young man's limbs, revealing his bones, his teeth to rot, his breath to stink and his voice to fail.

Fracastoro noted that the disease appeared simultaneously in many countries, doubting the popular theory that it came from America brought back to Europe with Columbus's sailors. It is likely that syphilis has always existed in the Old World, and that the causative organism, *Treponema pallidum*, underwent a world-wide mutation at the close of the fifteenth century, attacking previously resistant hosts in the Orient as well as in Europe. Mediaeval medical writings refer to cases of venereal leprosy, probably cutaneous syphilis, which was treated with mercury then as in the 1500s. Besides, there are a few undoubted descriptions of the disease in tracts written before 1492.

Right: an early engraving showing the use of the tobacco plant as a treatment for syphilis, from a book on Brazil published in 1558. The central figure is an American Indian who is suffering from syphilis; he is held on the left and right by two people who are sucking poison from his skin. On the left a man smokes a cigar as a curative measure. On the far right a man offers the curative plant.

Below left: a man suffering from syphilis, by Albrecht Dürer, showing in hideous detail the syphilitic's painful sores and rotting flesh.

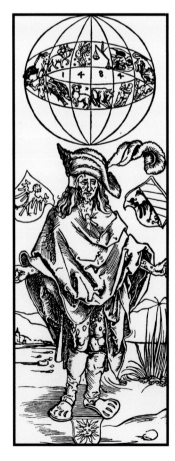

Perhaps commercial factors had something to do with the encouragement of the idea that syphilis had come from America. It is a common primitive belief that a disease and its cure exist side by side: guaiac, the 'holy wood', was used by the natives of the New World and was brought by Spanish sailors to Europe, where, in the form of infusions, its remarkable efficacy against the new disease was reported. Fracastoro and the German knight Ulrich von Hutten (who died miserably of syphilis) were enthusiastic about the new treatment, which was in fact quite useless.

Conditions then prevalent in Europe were all too suitable for the spread of syphilis. In Rome, when America was discovered, the town treasury collected over 30,000 scudos a year from brothels, and the historian Marino Sanudo estimated that Venice with a population of 300,000 people had 12,000 prostitutes.

If it is true that prostitution facilitated the spread of the disease, it is also true that medicine in the 1500s – in comparison with previous centuries – approached this plague quite differently. In particular, various prophylactic measures, effective to a certain extent, were adopted. The times were gone when an unknown disease appeared and a corner had to be found for it in the theory of the humours, instead doctors tried to build up a picture of the disease based on their observations.

In Paris, in 1497, the civic authorities issued an order under which all syphilitics not habitually resident in Paris were to leave. The Scots were among the first to become aware that the disease spread through sexual contact – a regulation made by the town council of Aberdeen stated that to protect citizens against the disease that had come over from France, women of ill-fame were to stop working on pain of being branded.

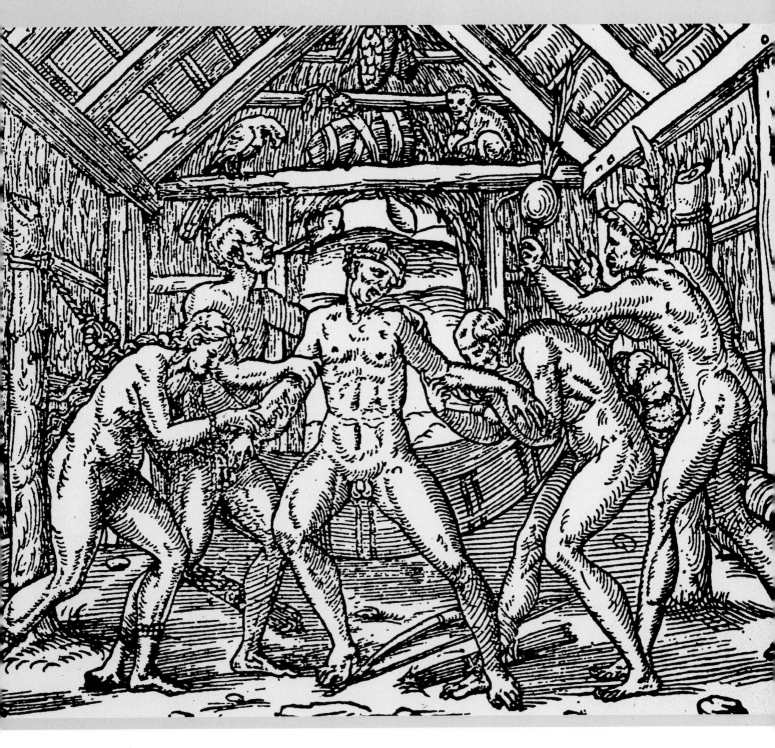

Leonicenus had described syphilis accurately as early as 1497, while Antonio Benivieni (1440–1502) observed that the infection could be transmitted from mother to foetus. Fracastoro was the first to suggest that invisible germs, which he called 'seminaria', caused contagious disease, distinguishing between poison (like snake bites) and 'live contagion' and noting the need to destroy the germs. 'Were it possible to destroy them with caustics,' he wrote in reference to tuberculosis, which he defined as contagious, 'there could be no better remedy' but as these substances cannot be used without endangering the lung, treatment can be tried through neighbouring organs.' Fracastoro recognized three kinds of contagion: one by simple contact; another by means of some carrier, such as clothing, bed linen or personal belongings; and a third kind by transmission, such as when germs propagated in the air and chose the most suitable spot to fasten on.

PARACELSUS

The spirit of the Renaissance gradually spread through Europe, although in 1500 no German university faculty of medicine as yet had more than two professors. The Silesian Johannes Lange (1485–1565) studied medicine at Pisa and on his return to Germany described the position of medicine and the 'ignorant and over-weening' medical men in his own land as pitiful.

The great English medical humanist was Thomas Linacre (1460–1524), the founder of the Royal College of Physicians in London and physician to Henry VII and Henry VIII. He studied in Italy and gained medical degrees at Padua and later at Oxford. Apart from his clear and accurate Latin translations of a number of Galen's works, which were widely read throughout Europe, and his foundation of medical lectures at Oxford and Cambridge, he also wrote books on grammar.

In France, a typical figure of the Renaissance was François Rabelais (c.1495–1553), like Linacre a priest as well as a doctor, who studied medicine at the famous university of Montpellier and then became physician to the hospital at Lyons. He also produced one of the first Latin translations of Hippocrates's *Aphorisms* and edited the works of Galen, but it is as the author of the cruelly satirical *Gargantua and Pantagruel* that he has gone down in history.

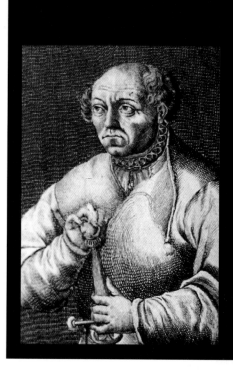

Paracelsus was the author of more than three hundred works, ranging from practical works on medicine containing much original observation to studies on alchemy and metaphysics.

The most notable German-speaking reformer of the Renaissance was, beyond doubt, Philippus Aureolus Theophrastus Bombastus von Hohenheim, the self-styled Paracelsus. A brilliant but controversial figure, he collected as many admirers as critics during his life-time but never seemed able to decide whether his main interest was natural science or magic, cabalistic knowledge and alchemy. He was well aware that medicine must forsake the teaching of Galen and start afresh, but he erred in his theory of the composition of matter from sulphur, mercury and salt. In the alchemical concept of Paracelsus these three elements were the outcome of distillation: the vapour condensing in the alembic was called sulphur, mercury was the scanty dense liquid remaining, while salt was the dry residue.

Paracelsus was born in 1493 in Einsiedeln in Switzerland, the only son of a doctor who went to the Tyrol when Theophrastus was nine years old. It is also known that in Austria Theophrastus started studying minerals and metals and that he was initiated into the secrets of alchemy and astrology by Abbot Tritheim of Würzburg. He travelled from 1517 to 1526, studying for brief intervals at Vienna, Cologne, Paris and Montpellier. He himself said he took his medical degree at Ferrara in 1519, where his master was Leonicenus, but documentary evidence for this is lacking. From his own writings it would appear that he had visited the Iberian peninsula, Pomerania, Poland, Lithuania and Russia, had been to the tin mines of Cornwall and Sweden, and had served as an army surgeon with the Dutch and the Venetians. People often expressed surprise that he could have written so great a number of works despite this continual travelling from one country to another. In answer to those who wondered about the sources of the extraordinary information of all kinds contained in his books, he wrote, 'I went in search of my art, often hazarding my life. I have not been ashamed to learn from tramps, butchers and barbers things which seemed of use to me'.

In 1526 his restless way of life changed. In that year Johannes Froben, or Frobenius, the Basle humanist and publisher, who had long been suffering from leg trouble, was advised by his doctors to have his leg amputated to save

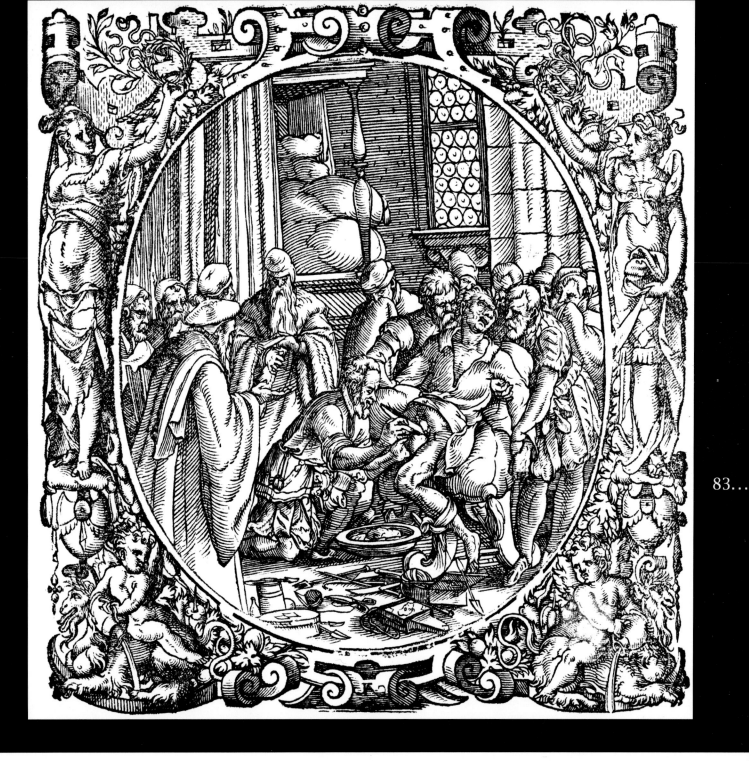

Above left: Philippus Aureolus Theophrastus Bombastus von Hohenheim, the self-styled Paracelsus. Apparently, he was given the nickname of Aureolus because of his golden hair, while his behaviour gave us the word bombast. Paracelsus came from his habit of prefixing 'para' to other words and is thought to signify that he rated himself above Celsus, the Roman medical writer.

Above: an operation for the stone, a woodcut illustration from Paracelsus's *Opus Chyrurgicum*, 1565. 'Very few surgeons,' wrote Paracelsus, 'have exact knowledge of diseases and their causes; but my books are not written like those of other physicians, copying Hippocrates and Galen; I have composed them on the basis of experience.'

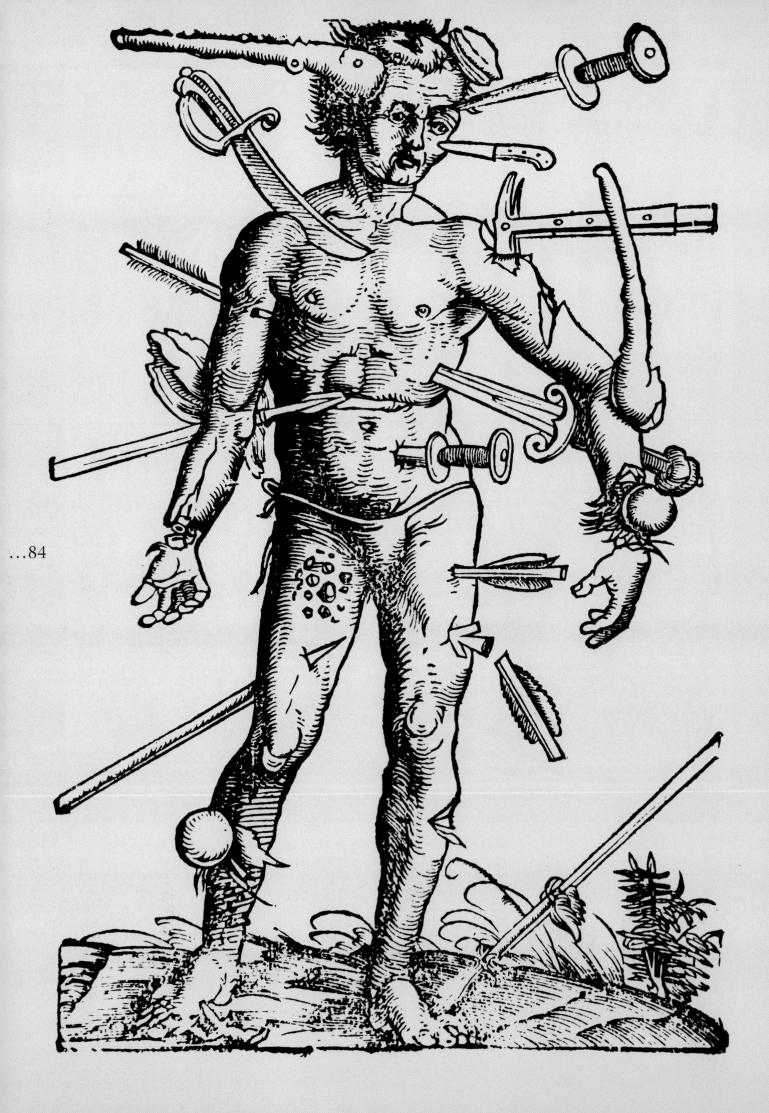

...84

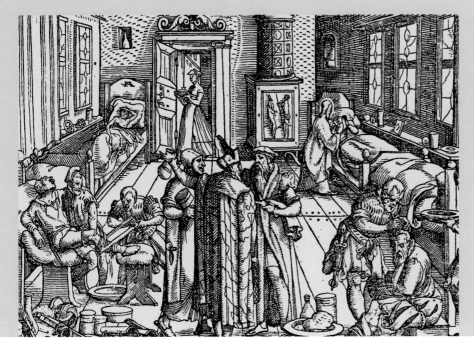

Far left: 'the wound man', an illustration from
Grosse Wundartzney, 1536, by Paracelsus,
showing injuries from different weapons.

Left: a busy ward scene, showing three doctors
consulting in the foreground and an amputation
being performed (left) and a head operation (right),
from the title page of Paracelsus's *Opus
Chyrurgicum*, 1565.

his life. Frobenius put himself in Paracelsus's care, and in a short time he recovered. Soon afterwards Erasmus of Rotterdam, a great friend of Frobenius, wrote to Paracelsus describing his illness and asking advice. The doctor prescribed treatment and Erasmus got better. It was probably on account of the reputation from these and other cures that Paracelsus was offered appointment to a university chair and as municipal doctor to the town council of Basle, an unexpected and welcome reward for a man who had identified with mercenaries and vagabonds.

85...

The speech with which Paracelsus made his debut at the university was characteristic and must have amazed his colleagues, who followed Galen assiduously and had never dreamed of prescribing commonsense treatment from their own experience. Paracelsus remarked: 'Thanks to the post offered me by the Basle authorities, which is an honour, I can proceed to teach students my methods, expounding for a two-hour period every day my precepts of treatment with the most diligence for the utmost benefit of my audience'.

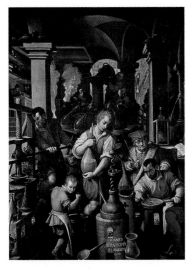

Above: An Alchemist's Workshop, 1570,
by the Flemish artist, Jan Stradanus.
Paracelsus took a keen interest in alchemy,
magic, astrology and cabalistic knowledge
as well as in natural medicine.

At the university, he broke with tradition by lecturing in German instead of the customary Latin and, even worse, he burnt the works of Galen and Avicenna in public, condemning the pusillanimity that for so many centuries had held back progress in medicine. To this act of revolt he added invective against his new colleagues, accusing them of propagating falsehood and thereby feeding the troubles of the world. After only two years, as might be expected, Paracelsus felt it necessary to leave Basle and return to his life as a wandering physician.

It is unfortunate that in his iconoclastic fury Paracelsus rejected the good things in the works of the ancient authors. Yet he upheld the Hippocratic principle that the place of the doctor was by the patient's sickbed. Paracelsus was a clinician in the best sense of the word saying, 'The doctor's character can influence the patient's recovery more than any medicine'.

During his travels he collected a great deal of useful knowledge. He was a chemical pathologist and a vitalist; according to the Paracelsian concept, the body's manifestations were subject to chemical and vital laws. He introduced the concept of metabolic disease and concerned himself with questions of hygiene. His admirable practical knowledge was shown in his works on surgery and his observations on syphilis and its treatment (mercury effective, guaiac useless). Through Paracelsus chemical remedies were introduced into medicine, and

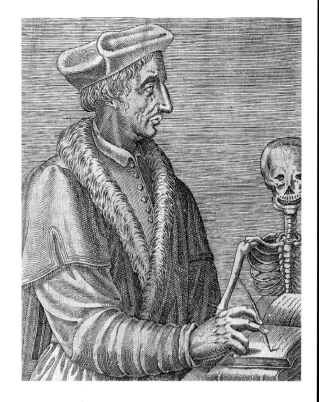

Right: Jean Fernel, professor of medicine in Paris, who was the first man to write a textbook on medicine. Apart from anatomy, it covered almost the entire field of medicine, but was strongly attached to the doctrine of humours.

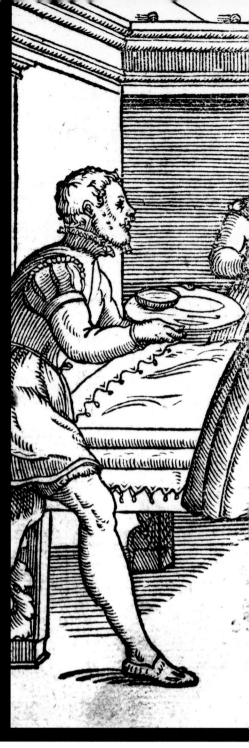

cine, and pharmacology began to make use of many new products. Paracelsus wrote a treatise on the diseases of miners, which may be considered the first work on occupational disease. He discussed diseases that 'deprive man of reason', and he recognized the connection between cretinism and goitre. He also wrote on epilepsy and the dancing mania. He died in 1541 at Salzburg when he was only forty-eight.

...86

The greatest contemporary of Paracelsus was Jean Fernel (1497–1558), a native of Amiens, who became professor of medicine in Paris and, while very much a man of his time, was instrumental in loosening the hold of Galen on medical thought and added a considerable amount to medical progress. He invented the terms physiology and pathology, and his writings, collected together as *Universa medica*, remained the standard text for the next two centuries. Fernel was the first to give a clear description of appendicitis and to suggest a syphilitic origin of aortic aneurysms, and he also observed something that Vesalius missed, namely that the spinal cord is hollow.

Girolamo Cardano was another brilliant man who led a stormy and turbulent life. Illegimate and a gambler, he was born in Pavia in 1501 where his father Fazio was a jurist and public lecturer in geometry in Milan, and a friend of Leonardo da Vinci. Girolamo attended the university of Pavia and then went to Padua, where in 1525 he was elected rector and a year later he took his degree in medicine. Because of his illegitimacy, he was refused admission to the college of physicians in Milan.

Cardano lived wretchedly for a while, but circumstances improved when he made his name with the publication of *Practica arithmeticae et mensurandi singularis* in 1539, and, in 1545, he composed the *Ars magna*, the most important algebraic work of the Renaissance, which contained the solution of the cubic equation (still wrongly called Cardano's formula).

Although involved with mathematics and philosophy, Cardano was also a great doctor. In 1552 he was invited to Edinburgh to treat the archbishop of Scotland, John Hamilton, who was thought to be suffering from a tubercular condition. After six weeks' observation, Cardano diagnosed asthma and recom-

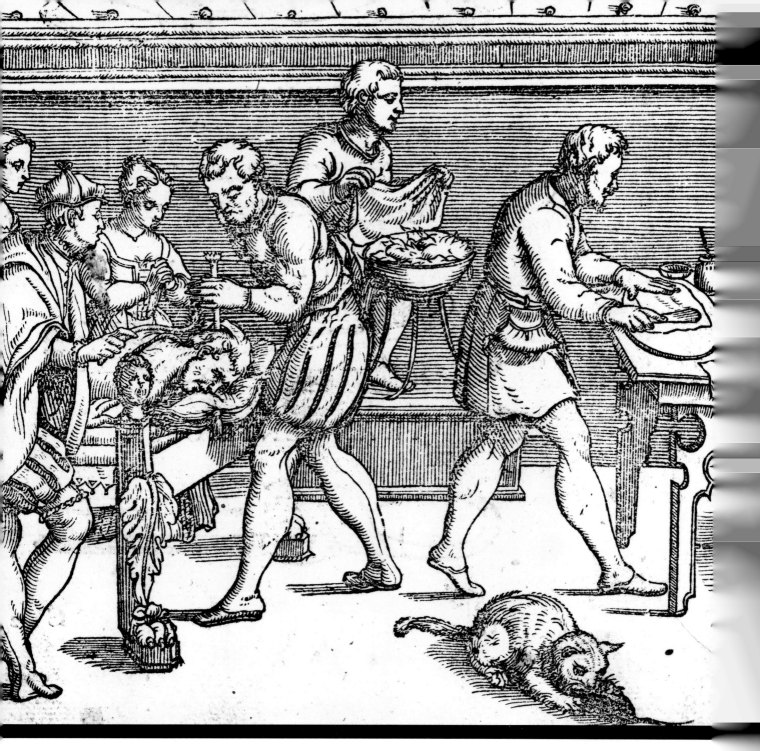

Above: a sixteenth-century surgeon performing a trephination, from *Cirurgia universale e perfetta*, 1583, by Giovanni Andrea Della Croce. Note the cat eating a mouse in the foreground.

mended that the archbishop sleep between sheets of raw silk and without feather pillows. John Hamilton recovered; it may be supposed that he was allergic to feathers. Cardano also devised a form of writing for the blind which anticipated braille, and a means for teaching the deaf to communicate.

Tragedy darkened Cardano's life: his son poisoned his wife, was sentenced to death and beheaded. Cardano wrote *De utilitate ex adversis capienda*, in which he described the psychopathic trait. He stated it was 'nothing but a disorder of the mind, a malignant doltishness, which does not show the signs of complete insanity, for those suffering it are able to exercise some choice'.

Felix Platter of Basle (1563–1614) was the first man to try to distinguish between various mental disorders: *mentis imbecilitas* (mental deficiency), *mentis consternatio* (loss of consciousness, and in epilepsy and in some strokes), *mentis alienatio* (psychosis) and *mentis defatigatio* (anxiety state). Platter studied medicine at the universities of Basle, Montpellier and Paris and was a follower of Vesalius in anatomy, although he held such traditional views as to believe melancholia to be the work of the devil.

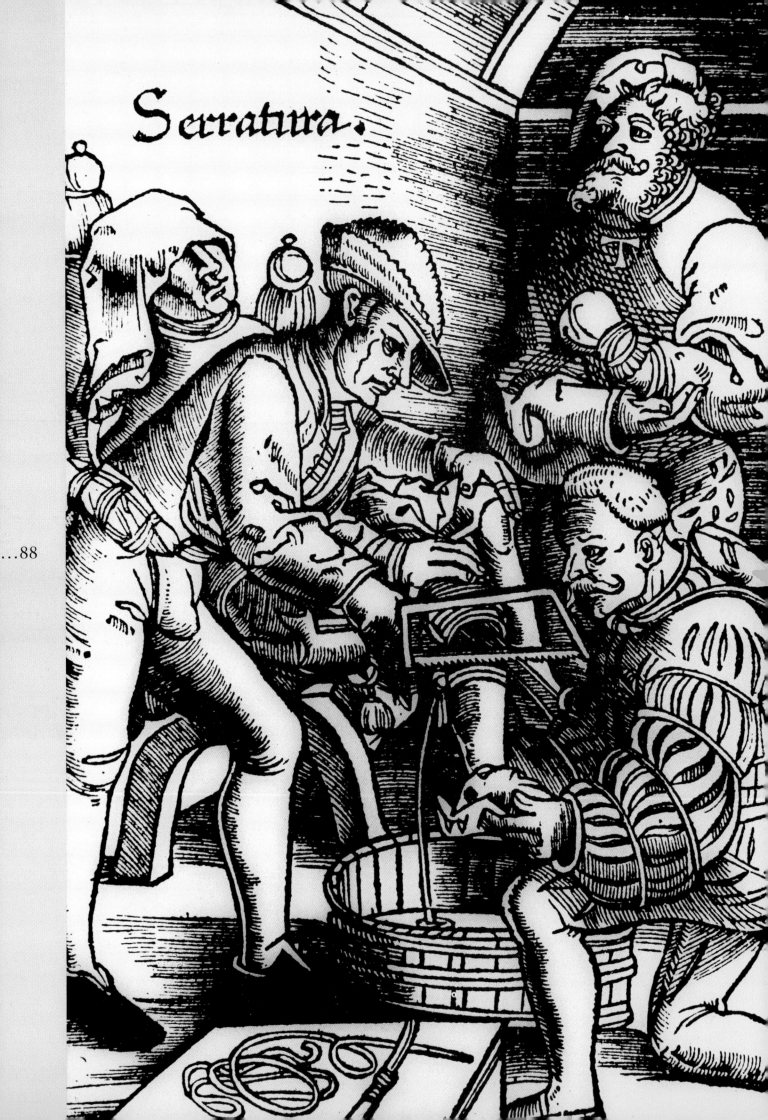

Serratura.

...88

PARE AND 16TH-CENTURY SURGERY

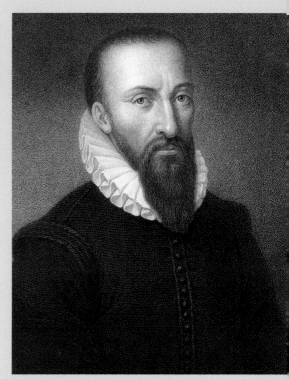

'In the year 1536, Francis the King of France sent a great expeditionary force to Piedmont to conquer Turin and recapture cities and castles . . . The soldiers of the fort, seeing our forces launching an all-out attack, did their best to defend themselves and killed and wounded many with all types of weapons but chiefly gunshot, so that the surgeons had a great deal of work on their hands. At the time, to tell the truth, I was still a beginner, never having seen gunshot wounds treated. True, I had read in the eighth chapter of the first book of Giovanni da Vigo's *Delle ferite in generale* that wounds caused by firearms were poisonous because of the gunpowder and that the best treatment was to cauterize them with boiling oil of elder mixed with treacle.

'Knowing that boiling oil was sure to cause the wounded terrible pain, before applying it I asked what the other surgeons used for the first dressing. It was only when I learned that they poured the oil as hot as possible into the wound that I summoned up courage to do likewise. But then I ran out of oil and was obliged to apply a mixture of egg yolk, oil of roses and turpentine. That night I was unable to sleep thinking I was going to find that my wounded patients had died because I had not performed the cauterization with boiling oil. So I got up before daybreak and went to have a look at them. What I found was beyond my wildest hope, for those to whom I had given my mixture felt little pain and their wounds were not inflamed. On the other hand, I discovered that all those to whom I had administered the boiling oil were in dreadful pain and with the injured part inflamed. At this I decided that never again would I burn so cruelly the poor men who had been wounded by arquebus shots.'

Thus it was a novice who put an end to the atrocious practice of burning wounds with hot iron or boiling oil. This beginner was the Frenchman Ambroise Paré (1517–90), later to become the leading surgeon of the Renaissance. The passage quoted reveals the honest professional, full of compassion for the suffering, intelligent and endowed with acute powers of observation and also lacking in knowledge in some respects.

Paré's father and a paternal uncle were barber-surgeons, the lowest level in the medical hierarchy. Surgeons formed the confraternity of St Cosmas and concerned themselves with the treatment of wounds, cauterization, the lancing of abscesses and the application of ointments and plasters. Major operations were entrusted to these modest practitioners, who besides shaving their customers used to let blood by applying leeches or cupping vessels. Paré, who had had little schooling, was ignorant of Latin and Greek and therefore unable to study at the university, planned to become a barber-surgeon.

A sketchy education became an asset, for Paré learned his art from first-hand experience, first with a barber-surgeon in Paris, then as house surgeon at the Hôtel-Dieu, a Paris hospital, and then as an army surgeon. It was through his intelligence as well as his lack of reverence for the old masters that he was able to abolish overnight the cauterization of wounds. In the tenth century Albucasis had advised the use of the cautery only as a last resort, but later it had come into indiscriminate use. Because of his opposition to the barbarous methods used on the battlefield, Paré became the idol of the army.

Above: Ambroise Paré, who as a young man put an end to the atrocious practice of cauterizing wounds and became the idol of the army.

Left: the first picture of an amputation, a woodcut from *Feldtbuch der Wundartzney* (the field book of wound surgery) by Hans von Gersdorf, 1517. The patient is blindfolded so that he cannot see what is going on.

89...

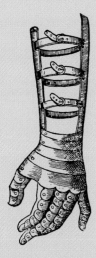

Above: an artificial hand designed by Ambroise Paré for the use of wounded soldiers, and in use from 1560.

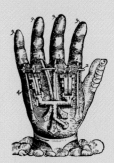

Below: another of the prosthetic aids designed by Ambroise Paré. Both illustrations are from his *Oeuvres*, Paris, 1575.

...90

'How dare you teach me surgery,' wrote Paré, the greatest surgeon of his age, in answer to a critic, 'you who have done nothing all your life but look at books. Surgery is learned with the hand and the eye. And you – mon petit maître – all you know is how to talk your head off, sitting comfortably in your chair.'

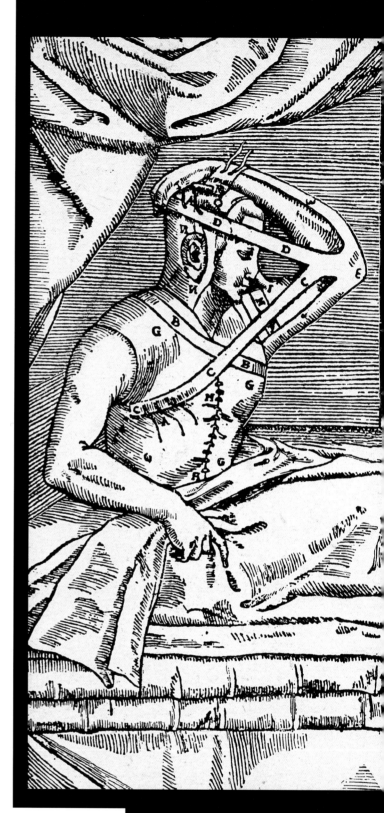

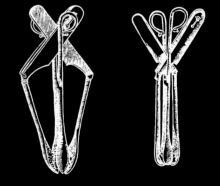

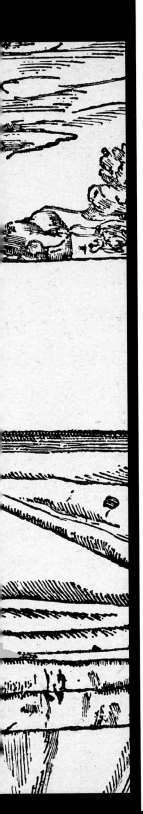

Paré also made systematic use of procedures devised by other people but seldom adopted, for example control of haemorrhage by ligation of arteries, and operation for hare-lip. He devised new surgical instruments, including haemostatic forceps and was interested in the problem of cripples, for whom he devised ingenious artificial aids. He also wrote on obstetrics and the procedure of podalic version for abnormal presentation of the foetus. The humble barber surgeon rose to become a councillor of state and surgeon to four kings of France, Henri II, Francis II, Charles IX and Henri III.

That Paré eventually decided to start writing was due to the inaccurate statements committed to paper by a traditionalist, Etienne Gourmelen, who attacked Paré in a long diatribe, criticizing in particular arterial ligation. 'How dare you teach me surgery', Paré replied, 'you who have done nothing all your life but look at books! Surgery is learnt with the hand and eye. And you – mon petit maître – all you know is how to talk your head off, sitting comfortably in your chair'. Paré was already famous when he began writing, and he found pleasure in giving a full account of his experiences as a surgeon and in war. The completed text was entitled *Oeuvres de M. Ambroise Paré, conseiller, et premier chirurgien du Roy*, and was published in 1575 at Paris, in a magnificent volume of nearly a thousand pages.

In the first engagement during the Piedmont campaign a badly wounded officer named Le Rat was brought to Paré. The young surgeon saved his life; when he was asked what he had done, he replied, 'I treated him and God healed him'. This phrase, with its expression of faith in the healing powers of nature, was engraved on his tombstone.

Among the surgeons of the later Renaissance mention should be made of Gaspare Tagliacozzi (1546–99), professor of medicine at Bologna, who made considerable advances in plastic surgery. Plastic surgery had been practised in Sicily in the 1400s by the Branca family and by two families in Calabria, but they all regarded rhinoplasty as a family secret. Tagliacozzi gave his technique wide publicity: it consisted in restoring the nose with a strip of skin from the arm of the patient, who was strapped up so that the graft did not have to be removed completely until it had taken. He also performed similar grafts for repair of the ears, lips and tongue. However, he was opposed by the authorities, who charged him with impiety and prohibited his operation, which was revived only in 1822.

During this period Germany produced, among other notable figures, Georg Bartisch (1535–1607), the author of the first book on eye surgery, *Ophthalmodouleia*, published at Dresden in 1583, and also Fabricus Hildanus (1560–1624), who was born near Düsseldorf. Hildanus practised in Berne, having studied medicine in Italy and France. He carried out amputations with a red-hot knife; according to him this horrifying system had the advantage of reducing haemorrhage to a considerable extent. Hildanus was also the first to amputate above, rather than through, a gangrenous part, and to amputate through the thigh, but he advocated a curiously archaic magical practice in dealing with the wounds – the application of ointment to the sword or knife that caused the wound.

Above: rhinoplasty, or plastic surgery for the nose. an illustration from Gaspare Tagliacozzi's *Chirurgia curtorum per institutonem*, 1597, showing the treatment he devised. The authorities considered that Tagliacozzi was interfering with the works of God and after his death his body was exhumed and buried in unconsecrated ground.

Left: two winged instruments designed by Paré for extracting gallstones.

91...

OBSTETRICS

During the Renaissance numerous books appeared on the subject of obstetrics, many of them written in the vernacular. In 1513 the most successful of these was published at Strasbourg, *Der Swangern Frawen und Hebammen Rosengarten* (The rose garden of pregnant women and midwives) by Eucharius Roesslin (d. 1526), a physician who practised at Worms and later at Frankfurt. The *Rosengarten* was essentially a collection of Greek and Latin works on obstetrics, but rendered in German and illustrated with twenty woodcuts by Conrad Merkel, a friend of Dürer. The use of vernacular language and the inclusion of illustrations probably account for the enormous success of Roesslin's work; it was translated into several languages in numerous editions until as late as the eighteenth century. An English version by Richard Jonas, called the *Byrthe of Mankind*, was published in 1540.

One of the best known of all Renaissance medical works, and one which like the *Rosengarten* was republished in innumerable editions until well into the eighteenth century, was an Italian book on obstetrics, *La comare o raccoglitrice* (The midwife) by Scipio Mercurio, first published in 1595, the year of his death; it is notable for containing one of the earliest statements that Caesarean section should be performed in the case of contracted pelvis. Advances in anatomy and surgery in the sixteenth century had an important influence on the practice of obstetrics. Vesalius and all the other great figures of the time paid attention to the deformities that may occur in the structure of the pelvis and studied the mechanics of childbirth. Paré is regarded as one of the founders of modern obstetrics; his *De la génération de l'homme* (Paris, 1573) combines Hippocratic principles with Paré's own original observations and modifications, and recommends podalic version, a procedure which Paré was probably the first to put into successful practice.

The publication of practical books on obstetrics was matched during the Renaissance by the growing number of works on the subject of paediatrics, many of them written in the vernacular. The first English contribution was the *Boke of children* by Thomas Phayre (d. 1560), published in 1545 as part of his *Regiment of life*, a version of the Salernitan *Regimen sanitatis*, while the first one in French was Simon de Vallambert's *De la manière de gouverner les enfants dès leur naissance* (Poitiers, 1565).

An Italian work was *De morbis puerorum* (On the diseases of children, Venice, 1583) by Gerolamo Mercuriale (1530–1606), who was also the author of the first systematic treatise on skin diseases, *De morbis cutaneis* (Venice, 1572). Mercuriale also attempted to explain certain psychiatric conditions, stating for example that the increase in melancholia which he observed was caused by the life of pleasure and excessive luxury that more and more people were leading, tracing its origin to a disturbance of the imaginative faculties.

> Many of the medical books written during the Renaissance were written in the vernacular, rather than Latin. Some of the most popular were on obstetrics and paediatrics and remained in use for over a century.

Right: an ivory statuette, probably German, of a pregnant woman, with removable parts designed to show the internal organs. Models of this sort were intended for students.

Below: a birth scene from Roesslin's *Der Swangern Frawen und Hebammen Rosengarten*, 1513, showing a pregnant woman on a birth stool with two midwives in attendance.

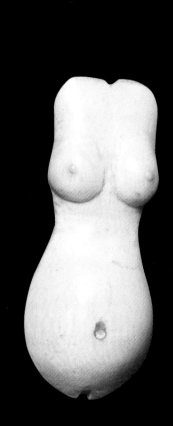

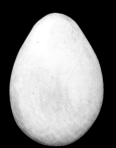

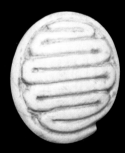

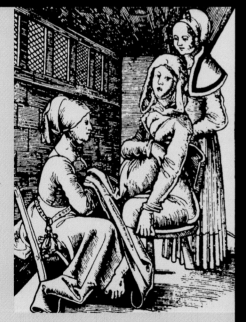

A GOLDEN AGE OF SCIENCE

In the seventeenth century the gulf between medical practice and advances in research was wider than at any time before or since. Medical practitioners were for the most part poorly trained and loath to keep abreast of developments; they continued to prescribe, whatever the disease, the same old remedies – enemas, blood-letting and purging.

When a new drug becomes popular, even today, it is often used enthusiastically and without every note being taken of side effects and specific indications for its use. This happened four hundred years ago with antimony. Although as a drug antimony was known in the time of Paracelsus, by the name of stibium, its fortunes only prospered after the publication, in 1604, of the book *The Triumphal Chariot of Antimony* by Johann Tholde, an alchemist, the author attributing it to a mythical friar, Basil Valentine. Tholde had observed pigs growing fat on a diet rich in antimony, and he applied this knowledge to treat a group of undernourished monks. Unfortunately the monks died. Over the next century violent controversy arose over whether this substance was a useful drug or poison. The argument abated when Louis XIV was cured of typhus after a dose of antimony. No one considered if the king would also have recovered without it, and so the substance became a universal panacea.

Another drug that was welcomed indiscriminately was quinine, introduced into Europe in 1632 under the name of Jesuit's bark, because it had cured the malaria of a Jesuit missionary in Peru. The Inca medicine man who administered the drug would not reveal the ingredients, and the Jesuit decided to find out the truth for himself; after a long search, he discovered that the remedy was the bark of a plant, the cinchona. The Jesuits held the export monopoly to Europe, earning great rewards from the acceptance of quinine as the cure that had been created alongside the disease.

Right: an illustration from *Catoptri microcosmici ... absolutam admirandae partium hominis creaturarum divinarum praesantissimi* (an anatomical representation of people in three parts, a sumptuous study published in 1613.

Below: the quinine plant, *Cinchona officinalis*, from Bergius's *Materia Medica*, Vol 1, 1778.

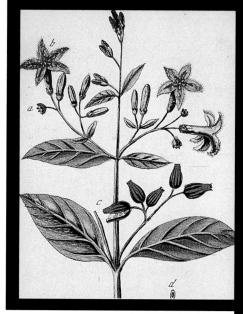

Soon after its introduction quinine started fierce arguments, because doctors were over-prescribing it in their ignorance of its toxic side effects, such as disturbances of hearing. Nevertheless its therapeutic worth was inescapable, and it had one other important effect, for it may well have played a leading part in the overthrow of Galenism. The Galenists held that the effective treatment of many diseases involved purgation, and while they could argue that the success obtained in treating syphilis with mercury was due to salivation being really only another way of expelling toxic material, there was no hope of explaining the effects of quinine in the same way.

Quinine was the great pharmacological advance in an era which clung by and large to the medicaments of an earlier age. Pharmacopoeias of the period included many recipes containing ingredients with magical properties – worms, foxes' lungs, lozenges of dried vipers, oil of wolves, moss from the skull of a victim of violent death, and crabs' eyes, to list but a few – and such treatments were prescribed by the leading physicians of the day. In addition many proprietary preparations earned fortunes for private individuals. One of the best known of these was Scot's Pills, a mixture of aloes, jalap, gamboge and anise, introduced in 1635 and still on sale in 1875. Baffy's Elixir was made up to the beginning of the present century, and the formula of Goddard's Drops, prescribed by Sydenham and said to be made from raw silk, was bought by Charles II for more than £5,000.

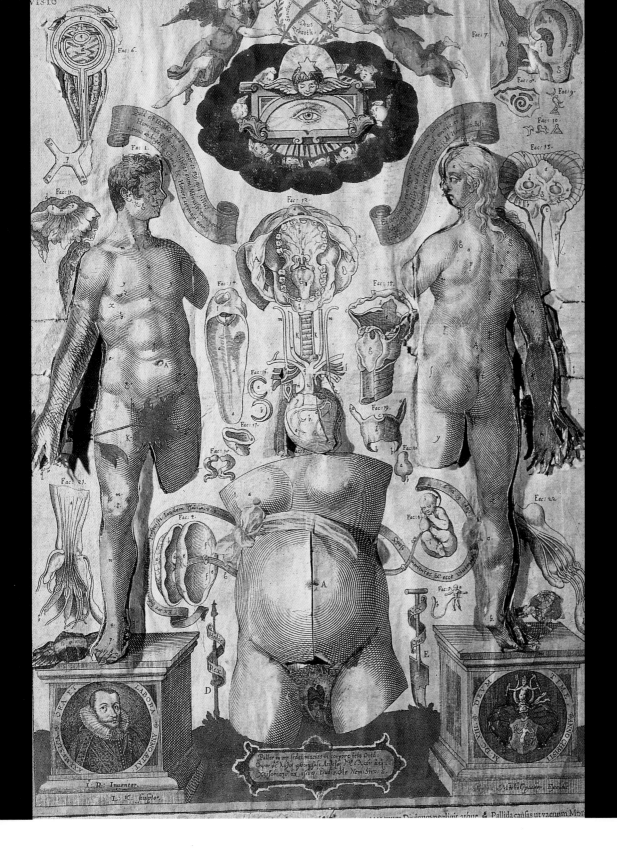

The seventeenth century presented a
paradox in that the natural sciences were
developing broadly and swiftly while
medicine seemed to be returning to the
attitudes of the Middle Ages.

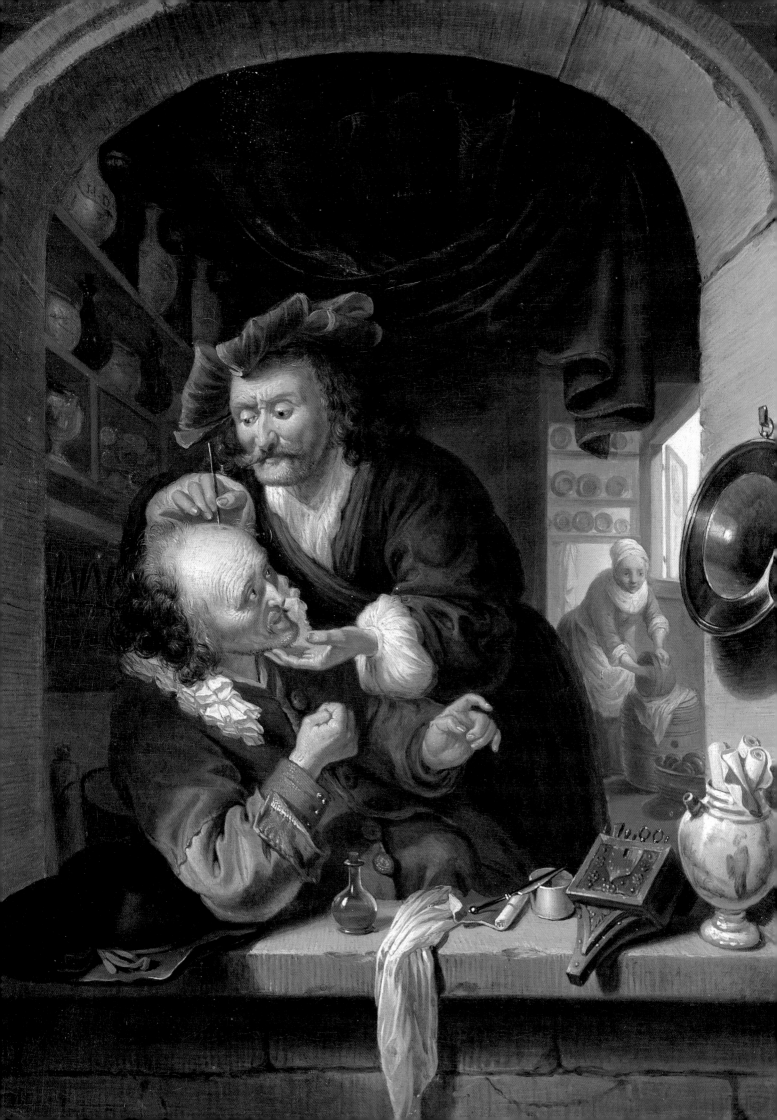

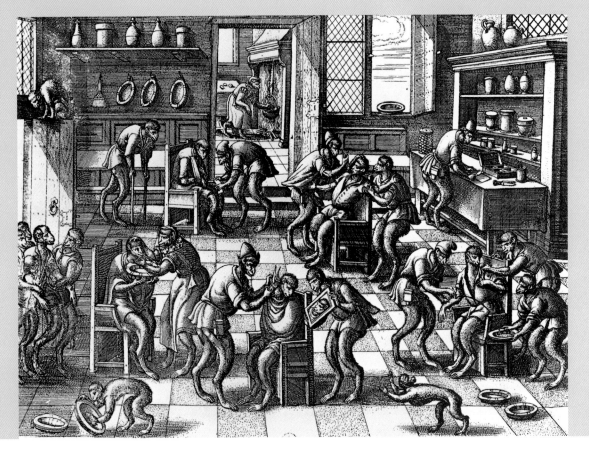

Right: a satirical study, dated 1570, showing a group of monkeys busy at their work as barber-surgeons, undertaking blood-letting, tooth extraction, surgery and hair cutting.

Left: The Barber-Surgeon by Issac Koedyck, showing a humble barber-surgeon treating a patient.

97...

These remedies and many others, some complex and some of the simplest formulation, formed the basis of treatment for a wide variety of diseases. Prices were often high, and apothecaries' bills were a source of dissatisfaction to patient and physician alike. Overcharging sometimes got out of hand: in 1633 George Buller asked for thirty shillings (£1.50) per pill, while a few years earlier the Royal College of Physicians prosecuted a Dr Tenant for charging £6 for a pill and a decoction.

The great progress made in anatomy in the latter half of the sixteenth century had surprisingly little effect on surgery in the seventeenth. Despite academic conservatism and the slow diffusion of the new knowledge it might be expected that surgeons would seize on the facts revealed by Vesalius and his successors and put them to practical use. However the surgeons, with the barbers, were still an underprivileged class, lacking a scientific education and far below the physicians in status. In England the company of Barber-Surgeons, incorporated in 1540, was allowed to perform dissections in its own hall, but not elsewhere. In France, the surgeon was regarded rather more highly, but he was still an inferior being. Guy Patin (1601–72), the dean of the medical faculty in Paris, showed his hate of his upstart surgical colleagues by describing them as: 'Mere booted lackeys – a race of extravagant coxcombs who wear moustaches and flourish razors'.

The position of surgeons, in France at least, was improved not by learning but by an event in 1686 which the historian Michelet considered 'more important than the work of Paré'. This was the successful treatment of Louis XIV's chronic anal fistula by the surgeon Felix. The happy surgeon was rewarded with an estate, a title and a fee of 300,000 livres, three times that paid to the royal physician. Thus at one stroke surgery was shown to be both a noble calling and an extremely profitable one.

Surgery benefited little from the great steps made in anatomy during the previous century and surgeons were still ranked far below physicians in status.

The seventeenth century saw a great advance in obstetrics with the introduction of the forceps by the Chamberlen family. The first practical instrument to assist childbirth was designed in 1561 by Pierre Franco, but in 1647 Peter Chamberlen produced a pair of curved forceps similar to those in use today. The family kept its invention a closely guarded secret, and with the forceps several of them acquired highly successful practices in London, earning large sums of money. It remained a family secret until after 1700.

The greatest obstetrician of the age was François Mauriceau (1637–1709). His famous textbook, *Des maladies des femmes grosses et de celles qui sont accouchées*, 1668, which contained the first accurate study of the female pelvis, was the standard work in several languages until well into the eighteenth century.

Although medical practitioners were still in the grip of formal preconceptions and were content with minimal knowledge, the seventeenth century was a period of considerable development in medicine. It was, in contrast, a century of the most grave economic and political crises in Europe, especially in Italy and Germany. The discovery of the New World and the Thirty Years War led, however, to the rise of England and Holland, which enjoyed economic prosperity and military power, especially sea power.

While literature and the arts flourished during the Renaissance, the

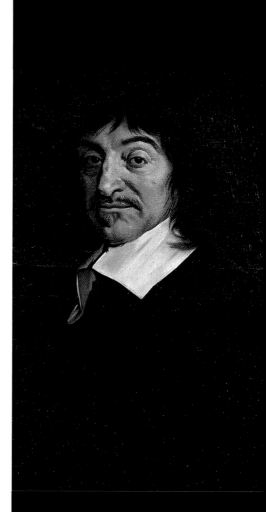

Above: René Descartes, Frans Hals's portrait of the French philosopher who believed that man was a machine except for the pineal gland, where the soul was found.

Right: The Dentist by Gerard Dou. In this Flemish painting of 1672, a dentist triumphantly displays the tooth of his unhappy patient.

The turn towards the natural sciences was inevitable in an age dominated by Galileo, who looked for an exact mathematical law governing every phenomenon, and Descartes, who based his philosophy on the concept that knowledge of one's own was the only absolutely certain fact.

seventeenth century was a golden age for science. The idea of Johann Kepler (1571–1630) that nature 'loves simplicity, loves unity and there is nothing superfluous in it' epitomized this era. The creators of the natural sciences – Kepler, Galileo, Descartes and Newton – stressed the need for direct study of nature in the light of objective criticism and without prejudice and dogma. In the new era of science, diligent and assiduous observation was the first requisite, with experiment as a test of hypothesis and with mathematical methods enabling a great variety of facts to be condensed into fundamental formulae.

The expansion of scientific research was not the only development to characterize the seventeenth century; another resulted from the fact that with Galileo science had become more exact. 'Science is measurement' is a concept which has influenced medical science not less than the other sciences, and one which medicine owes to Galileo Galilei.

The seventeenth century also saw the rise of scientific associations, the first of which was the Accademia dei Lincei, founded in Rome in 1603 by

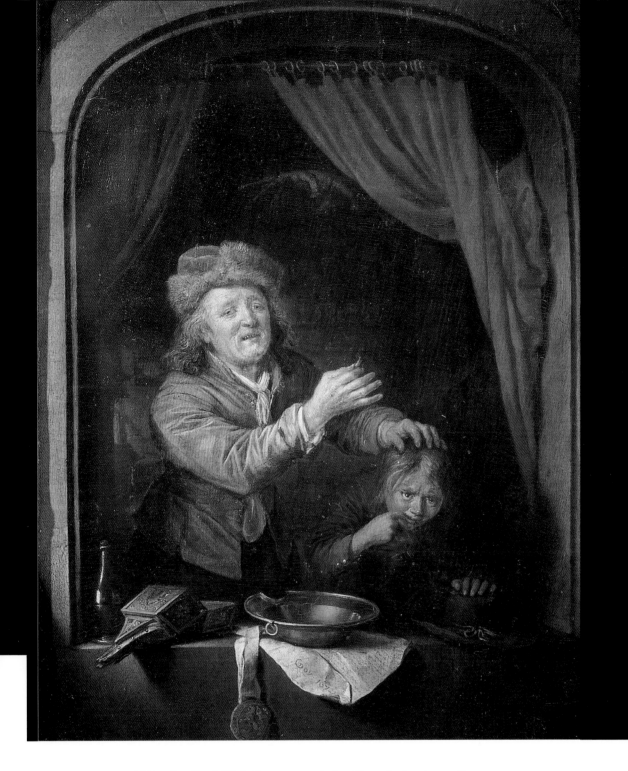

Prince Cesi. In 1635, Cardinal Richelieu created the French Academy. In London, The Royal Society was incorporated in 1662, and in 1700, Leibnitz influenced Frederick I to found the Berlin Academy of Sciences. The first scientific periodicals were issued in the seventeenth century. Medical contributions appeared in the pages of the *Philosophical Transactions of the Royal Society*, in the *Journal des Sçavans* in France and in the Venetian *Giornale dei Letterati*. The first medical review, entitled *Journal des nouvelles découvertes sur toutes les parties de la médicine*, began in 1769.

In the seventeenth century, therefore, medicine turned towards the natural sciences and experimental research. It was an inevitable development in an epoch dominated by the figure of Galileo, who looked for an exact mathematical law governing every phenomenon, and Descartes, who based his philosophy on the concept that knowledge of one's own was the only absolutely certain fact. A third giant of this era is Francis Bacon, who decided that a new approach should be made to the problem of systematizing knowledge.

HARVEY AND THE CIRCULATION OF THE BLOOD

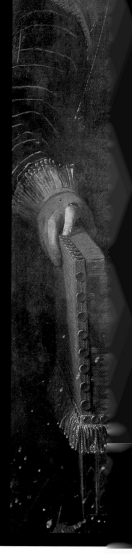

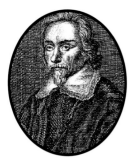

Above: William Harvey

...100

William Harvey was born at Folkestone in 1578; after studying at Caius College, Cambridge, he enrolled at the university of Padua in 1598. Galileo was a teacher there and without a doubt it was in Padua that Harvey's scientific method crystallized. Like other young men he was aware of the influence exercised by Galilean teaching; the atmosphere was one of freedom, and he learned from dissection and anatomical observation. In Padua he was a pupil of Fabrizio d'Acquapendente, the first person clearly to describe the valves in veins. When he came back to London, in 1602, Harvey married the daughter of Lancelot Browne, physician to Queen Elizabeth and James I; he joined the staff at St Bartholomew's Hospital and became a reader in anatomy and surgery. Meanwhile, he continued his investigation of the vascular system which led to his discovery of the circulation of the blood, which he announced in 1616. It was not until twelve years later that his classic work, *Exercitatio anatomica de motu cordis et sanguinis in animalibus*, was published in Frankfurt. In this book, Harvey described how arterial blood flowed from the left ventricle of the heart to the aorta and was distributed through this vessel to all parts of the body; having become venous, the blood was carried in the veins to the right atrium of the heart, from where it flowed into the right ventricle. This propelled it forwards into the pulmonary artery and from here to the lungs, where the transformation of venous blood into arterial blood took place. After passing through the pulmonary veins, the blood reached the left atrium and from there it returned to the left ventricle.

A number of Harvey's precursors had already refuted the Galenic doctrine according to which the liver was the centre of the circulation. The ancient doctrine maintained that the left ventricle of the heart contained air, or blood mixed with air, which reached it from the right part of the heart through invisible pores in the cardiac septum. Leonardo and Vesalius may have realized the truth. In 1553 Michael Servedo or Servetus 1715–53, a Spanish doctor and theologian, published *Christianismi Restitutio*, a work which earned him death at the stake for heresy. In this book, almost as an aside, he postulated the existence of the pulmonary circulation and denied the porosity of the septum, and in 1571 Andrea Cesalpino (1524–1603), physician and botanist and professor of medicine at Pisa, used the expression circulation in his work *Quaestionum peripateticarum*, and he obviously had some rudimentary notion of the existence of major and minor circulation.

Harvey's great achievement was to complete the solution of the problem, putting in a clearly worked-out form ideas which had previously been advanced without the backing of experiment; with great skill in the design and execution of experiments he was able to confirm his hypothesis. He suggested that the heart was a pump, worked by muscular force; he observed the phenomenon of systole, the contraction of the walls of the heart cavities at the moment when they emptied of blood, and diastole, the dilation of the cavities when filled, and with knowledge of the valves in the heart and veins, and the observation that veins swelled below a ligature, he was able to work out the direction of blood flow and so outline the mechanics of the cardio-vascular system.

Harvey showed that the flow of blood must be continuous and that it must always be in one direction.

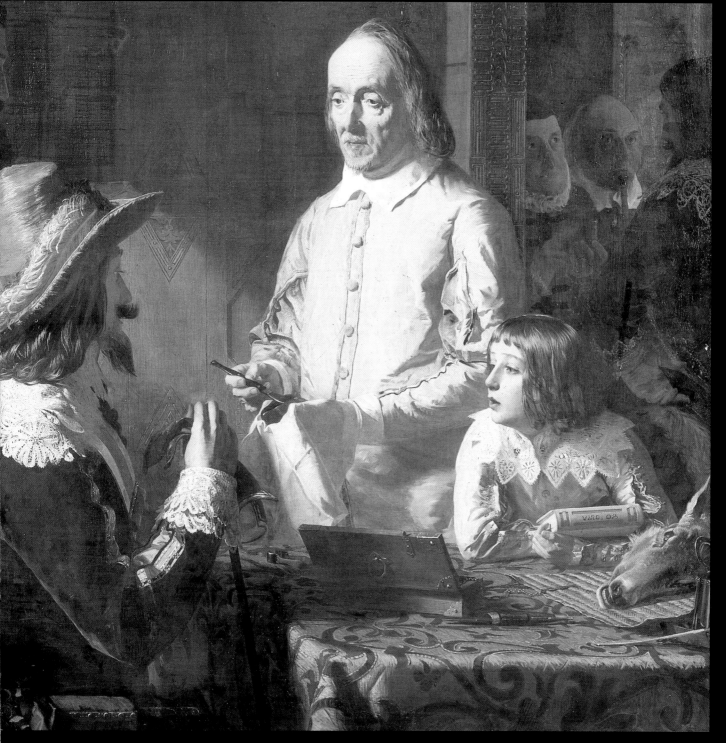

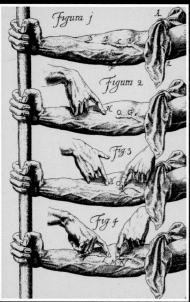

Above: William Harvey, who was court physician to Charles I, explaining his theory of the circulation of the blood to the king.

Left: an engraving from the first edition of Harvey's *De motu cordis*, 1628, showing the action of the valves in the veins.

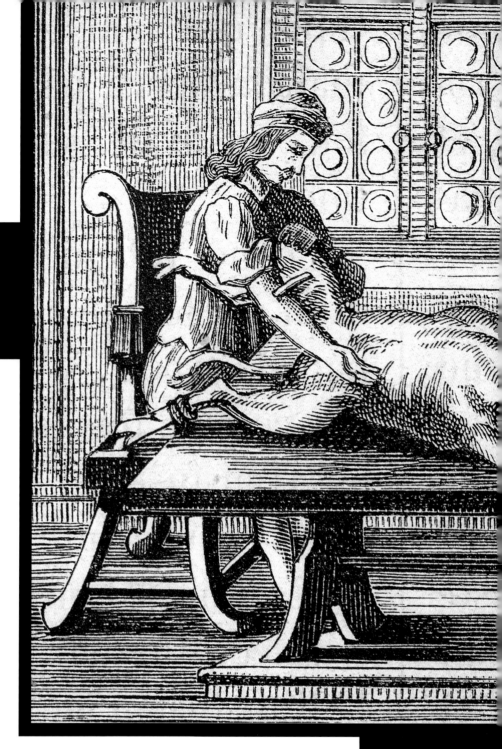

Right: direct transfusion from animal to man, 1679. The earliest description of a blood transfusion is given in an Italian text of 1630 but, despite the work of Richard Lower and others, there was widespread reaction against the idea of transfusing blood from animals to man, and the practice fell into abeyance until the early nineteenth century.

Harvey died in 1657, leaving behind him a massive epoch-making work. In the structure he created, the only thing lacking was proof of the existence of the capillaries; this was to be provided by Marcello Malpighi in 1661.

Harvey's other great work was published in 1651, six years before his death. This book, *De generatione animalium*, is of much importance in the history of embryology for it contained the theory of 'epigenesis', whereby the organism does not exist as a minute, preformed entity within the ovum but develops from it by a gradual building up of its parts. This theory was confirmed in the nineteenth century by von Baer, who had the advantage of the microscope; just as Harvey's concept of the circulation was limited to theory by one part, the invisible capillaries, so, without the microscope, his painstaking investigation of the embryo reached an impasse. Perhaps for this reason he fell into grave error over the nature of fertilization, which he believed to be something mystical, metaphysical and due to an incorporeal agent, likened by him to the magnetism transferred from one piece of metal to a second. This concept, as Garrison noted, contradicted the famous dictum '*omne vivum ex ovo*' by

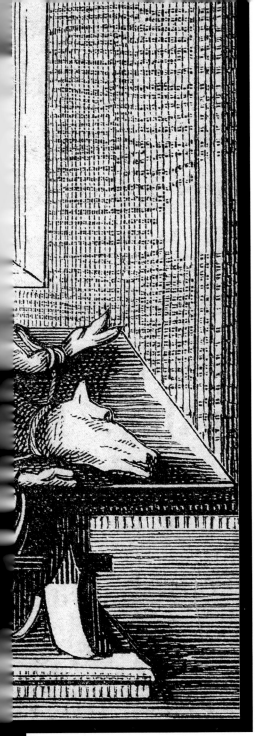

denying the continuity of the germ plasm, but was of value in Harvey's hands in that it went against the ancient idea that life arose from decay and putrefaction.

An important immediate result of the application of Harvey's experimental method to other problems was the explanation by four Englishmen, of the physiology of respiration. According to Galen, the purpose of respiration was to cool the heart, and the movements of the chest served to introduce air for generating vital spirits and to eliminate the smoky vapours of the heart. This belief was held up to Harvey's time, before when, as Allbutt wrote, 'respiration was regarded not as a means of combustion but of refrigeration. How man became such a fiery dragon was the puzzle.' A preliminary step in the working out of respiratory physiology was taken when Harvey showed that blood is changed from venous to arterial in the lungs.

The first advance came when Robert Boyle (1627–91) carried out experiments in 1660 and demonstrated that air was necessary for life as well as combustion, and that neither a flame nor an animal could survive in a vacuum. Seven years later, Robert Hooke (1635–1703), the pioneer microscopist, showed that by attaching a bellows to the trachea of a dog whose chest had been opened, the animal could be kept alive by artificial respiration and without any movement of either chest or lungs. Vesalius had done exactly the same thing over a century earlier, but now it was possible to say that the essential feature of respiration was not the movements of breathing but certain changes of the blood which took place in the lungs.

The next contribution was made by Richard Lower (1631—91), who was the first person, in 1665, successfully to transfer blood directly from one animal to another. In 1669 he injected dark venous blood into the aerated lungs of an experimental animal and observed its change in colour to bright red. He reasoned that this colour change must have resulted from some substance absorbed by the animal from the air in the lungs. Finally John Mayow (1643–79) showed in a series of experiments that the venous blood was made red by the addition of 'nitro-aerial spirit', a constituent of nitre (potassium nitrate) as well as air. Thus he came close to the modern concept of oxygenation of blood in the lungs. In addition, he advanced respiratory physiology by working out the function of the intercostal muscles, showing that maternal blood supplied the foetus with air as well as food, and asserting that heat production was from the muscles of the animal.

103...

Galen had assumed that there was a communication between the two ventricles through invisible pores. Later it was shown that the blood could only flow one way in the veins. Harvey put his own ideas into a clear form and confirmed his hypothesis with a series of ingenious experiments.

IATROPHYSICS AND IATROCHEMISTRY

By the mid-seventeenth century, the effort to free medical thought from the doctrines of the ancients was almost complete. The situation was fluid, with many new concepts more or less tenable. The genius of Galileo led to practical results, with the development of instruments invaluable in the service of medicine. Although unacceptable to pragmatic scientists, abstract arguments such as the mechanist theory of René Descartes (1596–1650) were also valuable.

Descartes carried out studies in anatomy, and immediately recognized the truth of Harvey's discovery. The author of possibly the first work on physiology, *Tractatus de homine* (1662), he envisaged the human body as a machine activated by the heat collected by the blood. The blood, sent towards the brain by means of the aorta, carried there the purest element, the vital spirit. The vital spirit dilated the brain and enabled it to receive impressions of external objects, that is sensations, and also those of the soul, which Descartes clearly distinguished from matter.

Iatrophysics and iatrochemistry, the study of physics and chemistry in relation to medicine, were born at this time. One of the founders of the iatrophysical school was Santorio Santorio, called Sanctorius (1561–1636), a professor at the university of Padua; he was the inventor of a clinical thermometer and an ingenious platform, bearing both his balance chair and his work table, which enabled him to measure alteration in body weight at all times. He thus discovered 'insensible perspiration', loss of water vapour from the skin. Santorius published the results of his experiments in a work called *De statica medicina* (1614), which anticipated modern studies in metabolism in its quantitative approach and use of precise measurement.

Another proponent of iatrophysical physiology was Gian Alfonso Borelli (1608–79), who taught mathematics at the university of Pisa. He attempted to

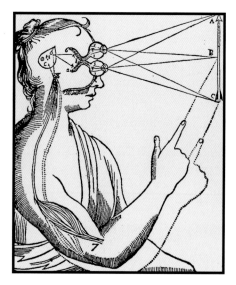

Above: an illustration from Descartes's *De homine*, showing the relation between sensory perception and a muscular action.

Right: Sanctorius in his balance chair. His experiments using the chair were carried out over a period of more than thirty years, and he frequently ate and slept in the chair.

Iatrophysics and iatrochemistry, the study of physics and chemistry in relation to medicine, developed during the seventeenth century. Descartes, Galileo, Sanctorius and Gian Alfonso Borelli were leading figures in the iatrophysics movement, while François de la Boë and the English Thomas Willis dominated the realm of iatrochemistry.

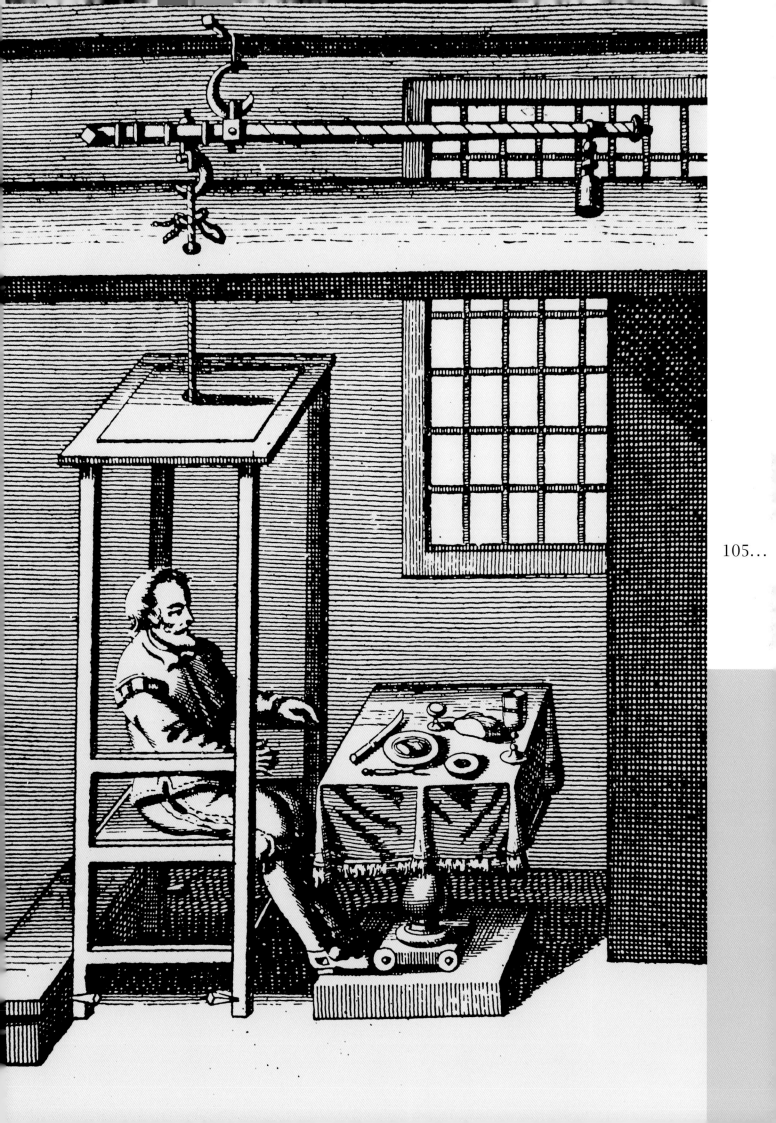

105...

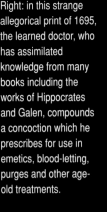

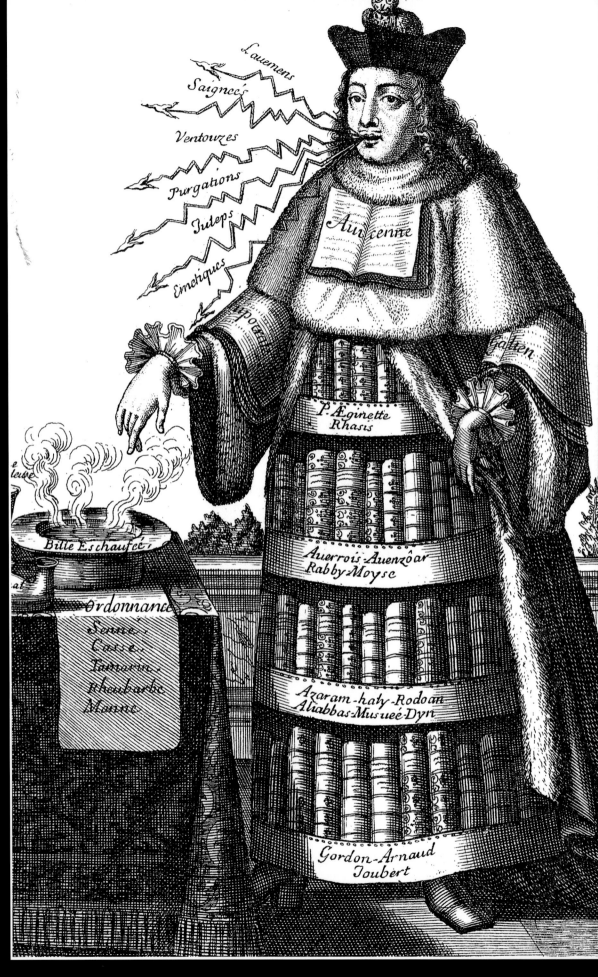

The mid-seventeenth century with its obsession with the measurement of vital functions led to the development of various instruments, including the thermometer, although it was some time before there was agreement on the scales to be used.

107...

explain the most important facts of animal life in mechanical terms and expounded his principles in a great work, *De motu animalium* (1679). Borelli studied the mechanical principles of muscular action and tried to measure the quantity of energy expended in movement. He affirmed that the volume of the muscles increased during contraction through the afflux of a hypothetical substance which he called *succeus nerveus* (nerve juice). When Borelli explained the respiratory mechanism he made valid observations on the function of the intercostal muscles and the diaphragm in breathing, but some of his other theories belong to the realms of fantasy.

The iatrochemical school was founded by François de la Boë (1614–72), better known as Franciscus Sylvius, a Frenchman who lived most of his life at Leiden in Holland. He asserted that all physiological phenomena could be explained in chemical terms. Pupils came to Leiden from all over Europe to attend his classes. One of his virtues as a teacher lay in his revival of the old custom of Hippocrates, that is of instruction at the patient's bedside. In a way, the school that he founded could be said to have survived him today; many researchers believe that life can be created in the laboratory.

Iatrochemistry flourished in France, Germany and particularly England, where its chief exponent was Thomas Willis (1621–75), a member of the Oxford group, which included Boyle, Hooke, Lower and Mayow as well as Sir Christopher Wren, who experimented in introducing food and drugs by intravenous injection.

Willis was born in Wiltshire, the son of a farmer, and graduated from Christ Church, Oxford, in 1639. He was professor of natural philosophy at the university in 1660 and six years later he moved to London, where he acquired the largest fashionable practice of his day. A fine clinical observer; he was the first to notice the characteristic sweetish taste of diabetic urine (1670), to describe the disease now called myasthenia gravis (1671) and to describe and name puerperal fever. He also made the original observation that some deaf people could hear in the presence of noise (paracusis Willisii) and produced works on nervous diseases, including general paralysis (1667) and on hysteria (1670). Today Willis is known best for his work on the anatomy of the nervous system, and his *Cerebri anatome* (1664), with illustrations by Wren, was the best book that had yet been written on the subject. It classified the cranial nerves, in an account which was accepted until the end of the next century, describing for the first time the eleventh or spinal accessory nerve (the nerve of Willis) and the group of communicating arteries at the base of the brain, which are known as the circle of Willis.

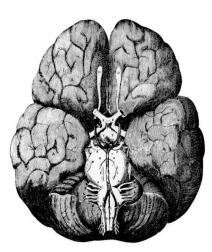

Above: the blood supply to the brain. One of Sir Christopher Wren's illustrations to Thomas Willis's book *Cerebri Anatome*, 1664. It shows the arrangement of blood vessels at the base of the brain known as 'the circle of Willis'.

THE FIRST
MICROSCOPISTS

The quest for scientific knowledge necessitated new instruments. The unaided eye, however keen, could no longer see enough. It was necessary to multiply its power in order to unveil the secrets of nature, from the most gigantic to the smallest. Most probably the instrument was invented in 1590 by Johannes and Zacharius Jansen of Middelburg in Holland. In 1610, Galileo was successful in adapting the telescope to focus on small objects, and the instrument was afterwards considerably modified by van Leeuwenhoek.

The man who worked out basic microscopical technique and discovered many new facts about man, animals and plants was Marcello Malpighi (1628–94). After studying medicine at Bologna, he taught at Bologna and Pisa, where he gave Borelli anatomy lessons in return for lessons on mathematics and physics. In 1661 he added the final piece of evidence to Harvey's work on the circulation by direct observation of blood in the capillaries:

...108

Right: Malpighi's drawings of a chick embryo from *On the Formation of the Chick in the Egg*, 1686. No 46 shows the whole embryonic area at two days, 47 is the embryo alone, 48 is the enlarged heart region and 49 is part of the segmented vertebral column.

Malpighi is known as the founder of the microscopic anatomy of living tissues. His work on the capilliaries completed the discovery of the circulation of the blood.

'I saw the blood, flowing in minute streams through the arteries, in the manner of a flood, and I might have believed that the blood itself escaped into an empty space and was collected up again by a gaping vessel, but an objection to the view was afforded by the movement of the blood being tortuous and scattered in different directions and by its being united again in a definite path. My doubt was changed to certainty by the dried lung of a frog which to a marked degree had preserved the redness of the blood in very tiny tracts, which were afterwards found to be vessels, where by the help of a glass I saw not scattered points but vessels joined together in a ring-like fashion. And such is the wandering of these vessels as they proceed from the vein on this side and the artery on the other that they do not keep a straight path but appear to form a network joining the two vessels. Thus it was clear that the blood flowed along sinuous vessels and did not empty into spaces, but was always contained within vessels, the paths of which produced its dispersion.'

But Malpighi's discoveries did not stop there. He was the first man to see red blood corpuscles, and he also discovered the papillae of the tongue, the intestinal glands, and the pulmonary alveoli. In addition, he made a detailed study of the microscopic structure of the skin, spleen and kidneys, and some of his findings, such as the Malpighian layer of the skin and the Malpighian bodies in the spleen, commemorate his name.

Marcello Malpighi did not have an easy life. His conservative colleagues at the university of Bologna waged a bitter war with him. Two of them attacked him in disguise at his home, while the anatomy professors insulted him in public and warned students not to practise dissection, on the ground that it was

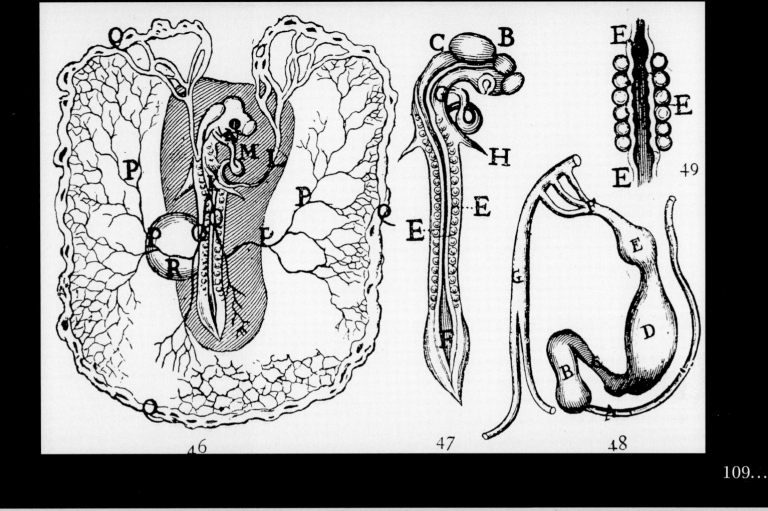

superfluous since Galen had already revealed all the secrets of the human frame. It seems incredible that halfway through the seventeenth century some university teachers still rigidly upheld the old doctrines.

Obscurantism could not prevail in the long run. The teaching of Malpighi bore rich fruit and was immediately acknowledged outside Italy. His work *Dell'anatomia delle piante* (On the anatomy of plants) was published by the Royal Society in London.

While Malpighi was making his discoveries, Father Athanasius Kircher, a German exile living in Rome as a result of the Thirty Years War, was verifying and confirming by means of the microscope the truth grasped by Girolamo Fracastoro – that organisms affected by a contagious disease contained minute, invisible living creatures which passed into healthy organisms and thus reproduced the disease. Kircher believed that the germs were born of corrupt humours and that in turn they corrupted the humours of the new victims they overcame.

A pioneer of the microscope whose contribution to science was of inestimable value was an amateur. Antoni van Leeuwenhoek (1612–1723), a Dutch draper who never left his native Delft, is considered the father of protozoology and bacteriology. He was self-taught and knew no Latin or Greek or indeed any language apart from Dutch. He began to use the lens in his business for counting threads of fabric, and built microscopes for pleasure, grinding the simple biconvex lenses himself and mounting them between two metal plates. He made over four hundred microscopes, continually improving the apparatus and achieving up to two hundred times magnification.

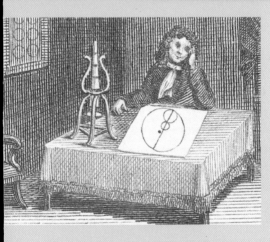

Above: Antoni van Leeuwenhoek, the Dutch draper and self-taught microscopist, whose intelligence and boundless curiosity led him to many original observations. By discovering the minute organisms called infusoria he initiated the science of microbiology.

In 1676 he initiated microbiology by discovering infusoria – microscopic ciliate organisms. Many people were indignant at this discovery, seeing it as further evidence of the perverted taste of scientists in attacking the dignity of man. Van Leeuwenhoek wrote that once he was astounded to see graceful little animals, more numerous than all the people of the Low Countries, when he examined a piece of food found between his own teeth.

Van Leeuwenhoek discovered a new world: protozoa, bacteria of various kinds, and spermatozoa, which for a 150 years were regarded as infusoria, their true nature being unknown. He also confirmed the capillary circulation discovered by Malpighi, observing it in the tail of a tadpole. 'When I examined the tail of this creature', van Leeuwenhoek wrote, 'I beheld the most exhilarating sight imaginable. While the tadpole was still in the water, allowing me to examine him at my ease with the microscope, I noticed more than fifty points of circulation of the blood. Thus I was able to state that the blood was conveyed through minute vessels from the centre to the sides of the tail, and also that each of these had curves and loops and carried the blood towards the centre of the tail for re-admission to the heart. It made me clearly appreciate this: the blood vessels observed by me are divided into veins and arteries, but in practice it comes to the same thing: they are called arteries when they convey the blood to the furthest parts and veins when they bring it back to the heart.'

Van Leeuwenhoek did not write books but his discoveries received wide publicity through the anatomist Regnier de Graaf (1641–73), famous himself for the discovery of the ovarian follicles bearing his name, and for his work on the pancreas and genital organs. De Graaf informed the Royal Society in London about the work of his friend the microscopist, and from 1673 onwards van Leeuwenhoek communicated his observations to the Royal Society in the form of letters, which were published at Leiden in four volumes in 1722. Thus he became celebrated in his own lifetime and was visited by many famous people, including Tsar Peter the Great of Russia.

During his visit to the Low Countries, Peter the Great also went to visit the anatomist Frederik Ruysch (1638–1731), who had made a famous collection of anatomical preparations, including several complete corpses or 'mummies'. The Tsar bought part of the collection for use in teaching anatomy at St Petersburg.

By this time, dissection had become established as a means of studying and teaching anatomy, especially in Holland, France and Italy; in England and Germany, where most material for dissection was obtained by grave-robbers (with the full knowledge of the anatomists), the practice still aroused some public apprehension and opposition. This period was also the heyday of Dutch painting, and doctors and dissections became a favourite subject of many of the great masters. Perhaps the most famous of these works is The Anatomy Lesson by Rembrandt, which portrays Dr Nicholas Tulp, professor of anatomy at Amsterdam, with his pupils.

...110

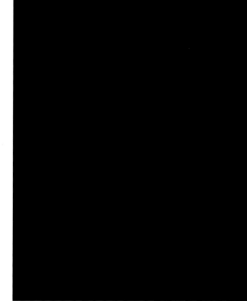

Right: Rembrandt's The Anatomy Lesson of Dr Nicholas Tulp, 1632, one of the most famous pictures from Holland's golden age of painting.

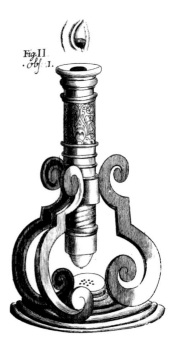

Above: a microscope of the 1680s, from Johann Franciscus Griendelius's *Micrographica nova*, Nuremberg, 1687.

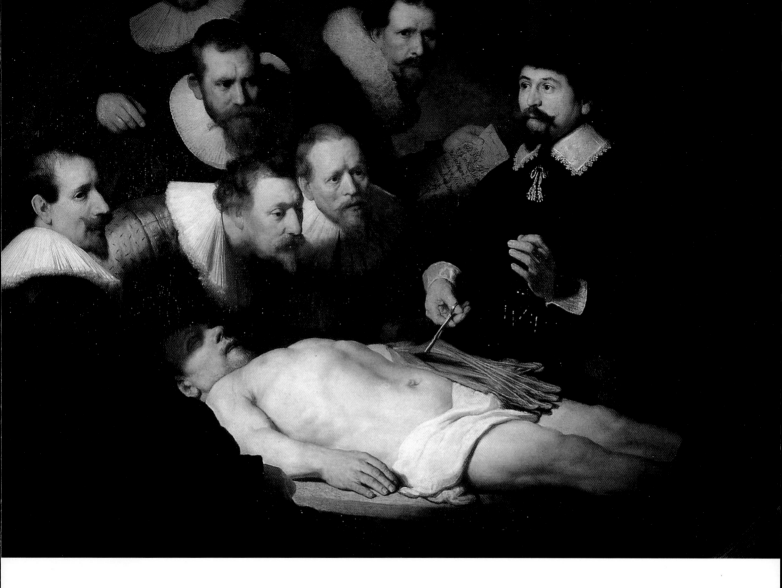

'I have often heard it said,' wrote Van Leeuwenhoek, 'that my reports are sheer fantasy . . . It seems that in France someone has actually said that the minute creatures described by me are inanimate. Yet I have shown the opposite to many eminent scholars and I dare add that persons foolhardy enough to make such statements do not yet have the experience necessary to pass judgment.'

SYDENHAM, THE ENGLISH HIPPOCRATES

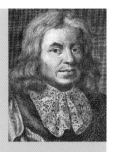

Above: Thomas Sydenham, a compassionate doctor with enormous commonsense.

Medicine was now advancing; the discipline of the exact sciences created the environment for future victories over disease. On the other hand laboratory study, research and experiments tended to make many doctors forget about the sick. Thomas Sydenham could not have come at a more opportune time, for he incessantly reminded doctors that their primary duty was to get to know and care for their patients.

The brilliant career of Thomas Sydenham, who was born in Dorset in 1624, was helped by his having been a parliament man in the Civil War. He obtained his degree in medicine at Cambridge in 1645 'by order from above', after he had been at the university only a year or so. At All Souls he soon became a fellow, replacing one who had been 'purged'. Thus through a politically motivated injustice he had sufficient authority to launch his necessary campaign in favour of clinical medicine.

Sydenham was profoundly sceptical about the natural sciences and theoretical medicine, because he considered the human mind too limited to be able to deal with fundamental truths. This attitude was characteristic of Sydenham, who saw all issues in black and white.

'The English Hippocrates', as Sydenham was called by his contemporaries, was a keen observer, describing rheumatic fever and Sydenham's chorea and distinguishing between scarlatina and measles, and giving a classic account of acute gout. He left superb clinical descriptions of such epidemics as smallpox and dysentery. He was very successful as a physician, thanks to the keen attention which he paid to symptoms and the course of illness, without concerning himself with standard professional etiquette. According to Sydenham, disease was something extraneous to the organism, which reacted by attempting to eliminate the disease-bearing substances from the blood. Sydenham held that all acute diseases derived from the inflammation of the blood and he shared the faith of Hippocrates in the healing powers of natu... standing therapeutic successes can be explained by the i... quinine not long after its introduction into Europe, and opium which he devised. This was known as Sydenham... regarded it as an excellent treatment for heart disease.

The fact that Sydenham paid little attention to anatom... all the scientific advances of his time is irrelevant to his task, ... of re-establishing the dignity of the medical profession.

Another celebrated clinician was the Italian Giovan... (1654–1720), considered as a pioneer of public health, espe... gestions about reclaiming marshland. He also proposed a rad... study of medicine. Lancisi believed that medical students ... based knowledge, should follow long courses of study, and...

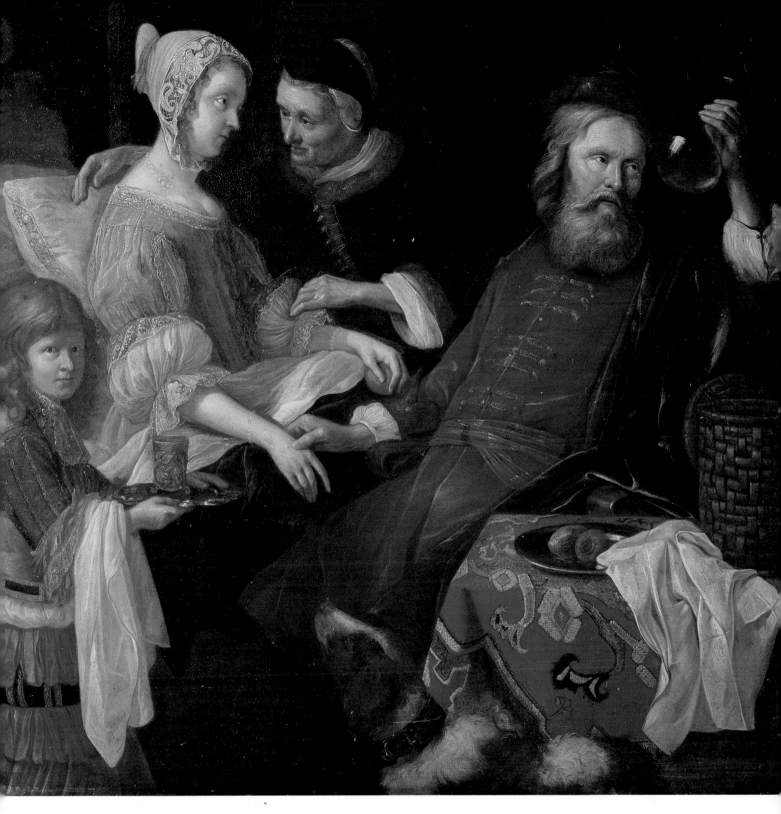

Above: in this study of physicians visiting a patient by Jacob Toorenvliet (1635-1719), one doctor is taking the patient's pulse while the other studies the contents of a flask of urine. Urine examination was still thought to provide a wide range of information, including the diagnosis of chastity and lovesickness.

Medical knowledge advanced considerably during the seventeenth century, but the profession's involvement with theoretical and experimental work tended to blind them to the needs of those suffering from the diseases they studied.

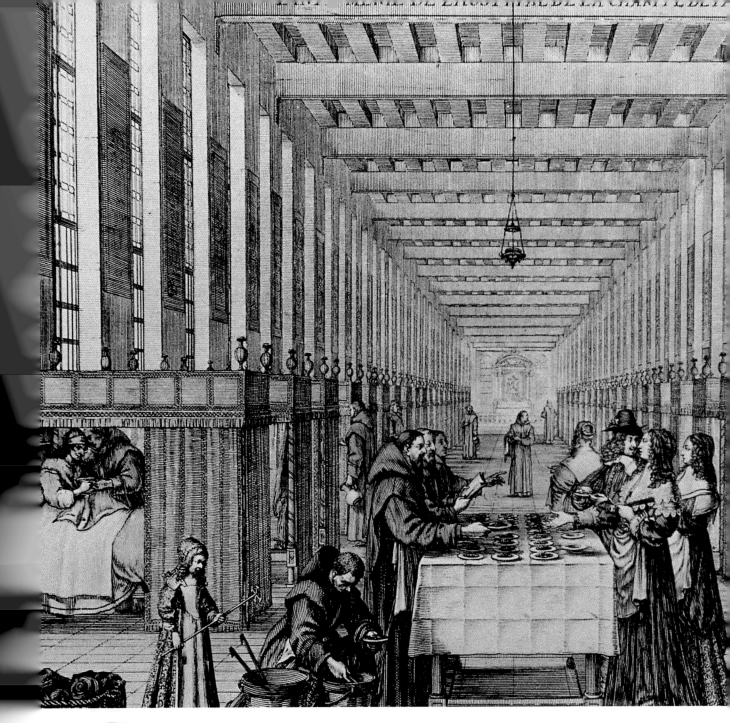

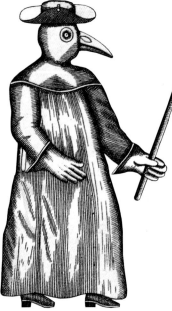

Epidemics broke out in Europe during the seventeenth century which were as bad – or worse – than they had been during the Middle Ages. Scurvy, in northern Europe, and malaria, in Italy, were rife, as were typhus, dysentery, smallpox and the most dreaded of all – bubonic plague.

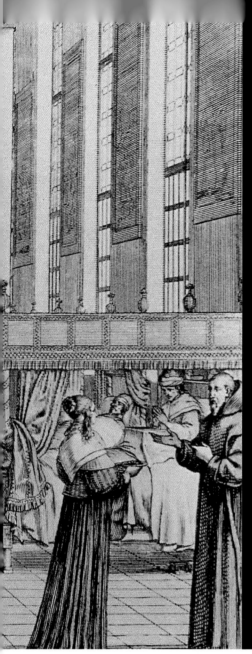

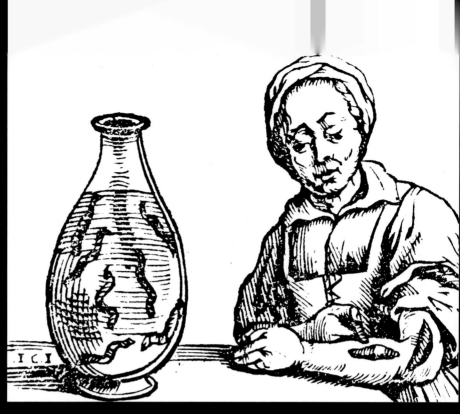

Above: men and women tending the sick and serving meals at the Hôpital de la Charité in Paris during the seventeenth century. An engraving after Abraham Bosse.

Above right: blood-letting with leeches was still a highly regarded treatment for many complaints. An illustration from *Historica medica* by Willem van der Bossche, 1638.

Left: the protective leather costume worn by doctors treating bubonic plague had not changed since the Middle Ages – nor had their treatment advanced.

themselves to anatomy and pathology and learn the use of the thermometer and microscope. At that period thermometers had come into use; they had been devised by members of the Accademia del Cimento and by Santorio, but no agreement had been reached about the scale. The modern clinical thermometer in fact dates only from the latter half of the nineteenth century, having been introduced into practice by Karl August Wunderlich (1815–77).

Another sort of medical instrument began about this period. The first book on vital statistics, John Graunt's *Natural and Political Observations upon the Bills of Mortality,* was published in London in 1662. The census may be a very ancient practice, but Graunt was the first person to establish, from bills of mortality, that more boys are born than girls, and that the population can be estimated from an accurate death rate. At this time there was no compulsory notification of births and deaths. Graunt's work was followed in 1695 by the Breslau tables of births and funerals compiled by the astronomer Sir Edmund Halley (1656–1742), which, by estimating mortality rates and the proportion of able-bodied men in a population, was the first scientific work in this field.

In spite of progress in medicine and improvements in living conditions, seventeenth century Europe suffered many epidemics as bad or worse than those of the Middle Ages. Scurvy was rife throughout northern Europe and Germany, malaria was epidemic in Italy, while in 1657 an outbreak of fever reduced all England to the state of one large hospital, according to Thomas Willis. Typhus, dysentery and smallpox ravaged the continent, and smallpox was also common along the Atlantic coast of the American colonies.

Perhaps the worse epidemics were of the dreaded bubonic plague – the Black Death of the Middle Ages – which returned with great virulence and claimed millions of victims, often reducing the populations of whole towns and cities by over a half.

Ineffectual plague doctors were appointed, who wore strange protective clothing, often all of leather – cloak, gauntlets and a mask with glass-covered eye holes, and a long beak filled with antiseptic substances, and carried a long rod to take the pulse.

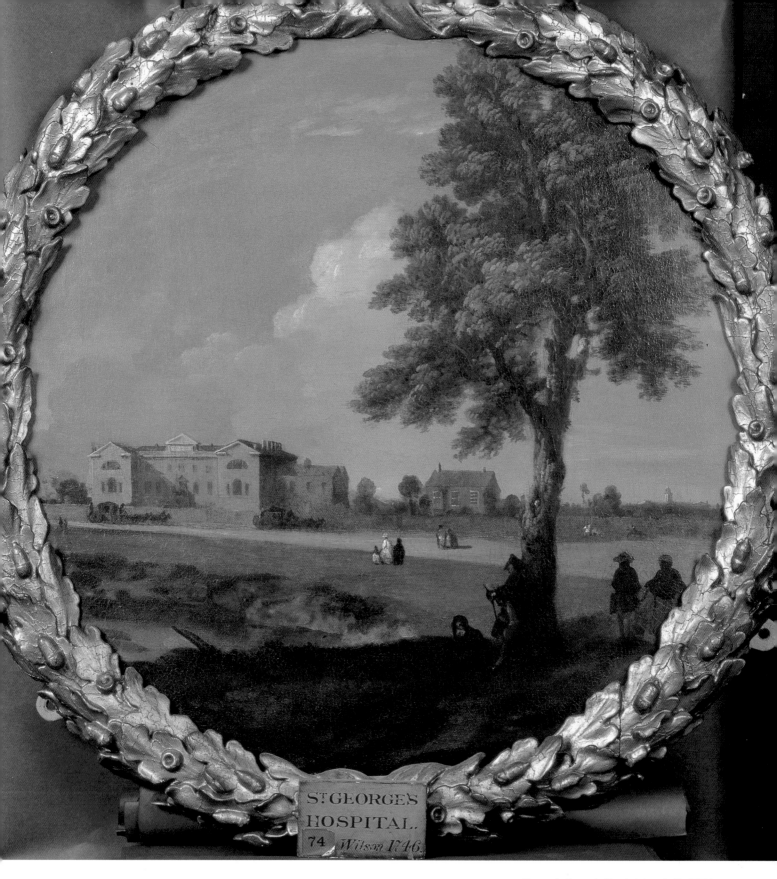

Above: St George's Hospital, founded in 1733 in a former country mansion, Lanesborough House, amid green fields at Hyde Park Corner, London. A painting by Richard Wilson dated 1746.

THE AGE OF ENLIGHTENMENT

The eighteenth century opened with the War of the Spanish Succession, saw the emergence of the United States, and closed with the French Revolution. It was a century of political upheaval and revolutionary idealism, which extended to all fields of thought and diminished the influence of academic dogmatism. It also saw the emergence of the physician in something of the modern style, his practice based firmly on scientific knowledge.

Eighteenth-century Europeans, besides looking increasingly inwards, came more and more to accept only what was observable directly and reproducible by experiment. This was a result of the increasing regard for the experimental method, the basis of scientific research since Galileo. There was considerable conflict between the new ideas and traditional trends of thought at the beginning of the century. On one hand there was renewed opposition to the experimental method, and on the other new ideas were gaining ground through direct verification of natural phenomena and formulation of natural laws. The conflict between the opposed ideologies ended with the triumph of the latter, and set the pattern of scientific thought for the nineteenth century.

The enlightenment that accompanied scientific progress had many direct effects on medicine and humanity at this time. Increasing awareness of the sufferings of those who were both poor and sick led to the foundation of many municipal hospitals and dispensaries. A number of the great London teaching hospitals date from this period, including the Westminster (1719), Guy's (1725), St George's (1733), the London (1740) and the Middlesex (1745).

Growing awareness of the sufferings of the poor and sick led to the founding of many municipal hospitals and dispensaries.

117...

The conflict of two opposed trends of thought led some doctors to oppose the new scientific attempt to influence medical doctrines by upholding animist philosophical concepts; this happened mainly in Germany, and could be linked in a sense with the Romantic movement. Other doctors, especially in Italy, vigorously opposed scientific mysticism and transcendentalism, and looked to new fields for explanations of physiological and pathological phenomena. It was through the work of Morgagni in particular that the basis was laid for the anatomical concept of pathology which itself was made possible by Malpighi's discoveries in the field of microscopical anatomy.

The trend towards systematic study was growing in many fields. In the natural sciences, the Swedish doctor and botanist Carl von Linne or Linnaeus (1707–78) devised a system of classification for plants and animals, and placed man in the order of primates with the name of *Homo sapiens*, in accordance with the binomial nomenclature he devised for all living creatures. Other systematic work was carried out by Caspar Friedrich Wolff (1733–94).

The old school of thought, however, gained new strength with the revival of animism in the hands of the German doctor and philosopher Georg Ernst Stahl (1660–1734), who declared that illness was a salutary effort on the part of the soul to expel morbid matter from the body. According to Stahl, the supreme vital principle was represented by the universal soul, which was the cause of every form of life and came direct from God. When the soul left the body on death the body putrefied. Illness was the tendency of the soul (which became identified with nature) to re-establish order in bodily functions. Stahl's animism was expounded in his *Theoria medica vera*, published in 1708.

Vitalism was distinct from animalism. It occupied an intermediate posi-

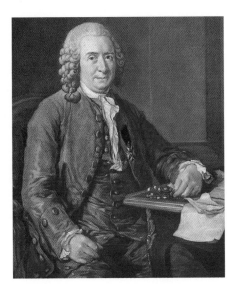

Above: Carl von Linne, or Linnaeus, the Swedish doctor and botanist who devised the system of classification of plants and animals known as the Linnaean system.

tion between the materialist doctrine and the spiritualist, and embodied the concept of a special principle distinct both from the body and the rational soul. The most notable exponents of vitalist thought in medicine were the Frenchman Theophile de Bordeu (1722–76), who taught that health was the co-ordination of the separate life of each organ of the body, Joseph Barthez (1734–1806), who introduced the term 'vital principle' and maintained that disease was each and every abnormality of normal function, and Philippe Pinel (1756–1826), the great reformer of psychiatry, pupil of Barthez, who anticipated Bichat in showing that certain tissues were subject to certain disease.

While Stahl was teaching medicine, botany and pharmacology at the university of Halle he had a difference of opinion with his friend and colleague Friedrich Hoffman (1660–1742) over the direction medicine ought to take. A fervent believer and rigid personality, Stahl was opposed to the materialism of his time, and pursued the aim of stressing the unity of the living organism with arguments that unfortunately were unacceptable to science. Hoffman, on the other hand, created a rational system on a mechanical basis and expressed his concept in a nine-volume work, *Medicina rationalis systematica*, published between 1718 and 1740. A follower of the philosophy of Leibnitz, he affirmed that our minds could not grasp ultimate causes and that our knowledge was limited to what could be gained through the senses.

All the energy of matter was conceived in terms of movement. According to Hoffman, life was movement, and especially the movement of heart and blood, while death was the definitive cessation of all movement. The human body was formed of fibres with the ability to contract or dilate under the influence of a nervous fluid secreted by the brain and distributed throughout the body through the nerves. The chief cause of disease was plethora (fullness), which acted indirectly through the stomach and intestines, at which therapy should therefore be directed. Hoffman's remedies derived partly from Hippocrates, but were partly of his own devising, for example Hoffman's Drops and Anodyne which are still to be found in some pharmacopoeias. Treatment of chronic diseases by 'tonics' such as quinine and iron originated with him and are employed to this day by some doctors.

Friedrich Hoffman was a modern scholar in the sense that he was in contact with colleagues all over Europe for the purpose of exchanging useful scientific information; he rightly believed that science was international. He was especially friendly with the Englishman Robert Boyle and the Italian Bernardo Ramazzini.

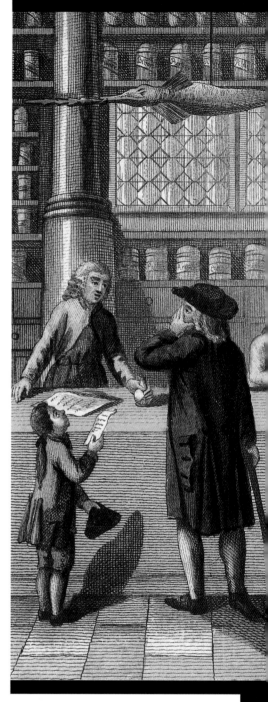

The eighteenth century saw the emergence of the physician in something of the modern style, his practice based firmly on scientific knowledge. Nevertheless, this was also the heyday of the charlatan.

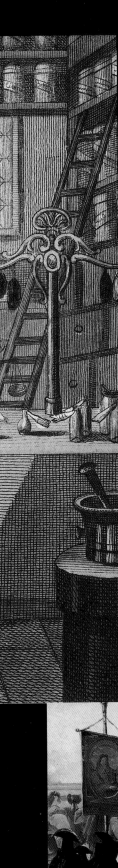

Bernado Ramazzini (1633–1714) who taught at the universities of Modena and Padua was the founder of occupational medicine. In his work *De morbis artificum*, Ramazzini systematically assembled his careful observations on working conditions and the causes of diseases in hundreds of trades and callings; among other things he noted the lethal effects of such metals as mercury and antimony. Ramazzini was not too proud to investigate the humblest or dirtiest work. 'On visiting a poor home', he wrote, 'a doctor should be satisfied to sit on a three-legged stool in the absence of a gilt chair, and he should take time for his examination; and to the questions recommended by Hippocrates he should add one more – "What is your occupation?"'

Hoffman should also be remembered for the importance he attributed to the nervous system in pathogenesis. William Cullen, the Edinburgh 'neuropathologist' also held that the nervous system regulated all the vital functions, and, in turn, his pupil John Brown (1735–88) produced a theory that life was ultimately not a spontaneous state but one imposed by continual stimuli: these might be internal, such as sensory perception, muscular contraction, thought and emotions; or they might be external, such as air, diet and atmospheric temperature. Good health was determined by an exact dosage of stimuli combined with normal excitability of the organs. In contrast, ill-health was caused by over- or under-excitation, as a result of some imbalance between stimulus and excitability. The morbid state could thus be sthenic, if the excitation were excessive, or asthenic if deficient. Therapy was a straightforward matter – sedatives for sthenic illness and stimulants for asthenic. The remedies John Brown himself preferred were laudanum and whisky. Though he died of alcohol at the age of fifty-three, his system – Brunonism – outlived him, for its extreme simplicity made it easily comprehensible and so had many followers.

119...

Left: an apothecary in his pharmacy, 1794. Since only the very rich could regularly afford the services of a qualified physician, those of more modest means turned to apothecaries for advice. A coloured engraving by Clemens Kohl after a drawing by Johann Sollerer.

Below: in Giovanni Battista Tiepolo's The Quack Doctor, the 'doctor' persuasively touts his wares before moving swiftly on to another town – and some more gullible customers.

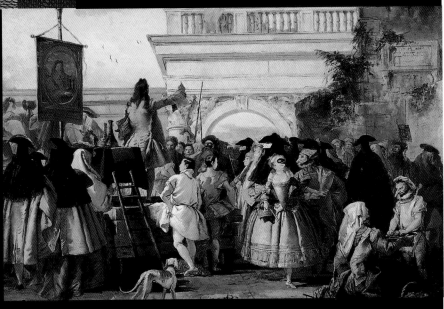

BOERHAAVE AND HIS DISCIPLES

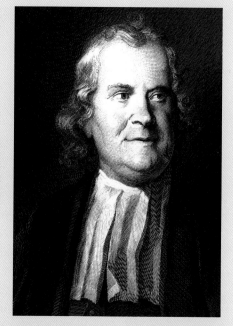

The outstanding clinician of this period was a Dutchman who acquired an immense personal fortune through his practice, and who was greatly admired not only by his pupils but also by the general public. This was Hermann Boerhaave (1688–1738). Boerhaave's classes were attended by students from all over the continent, and his published works, *Institutiones medicae* (1708), a 'physiology textbook', and *Aphorisms* (1709), went through a huge number of editions and translations into foreign languages, including one in Arabic.

Hermann Boerhaave was born at Voorhout near Leiden in 1668. His

Above: Hermann Boerhaave, who became so well known that he once received a letter from China addressed to 'Mr Boerhaave in Europe'.

The greatest physician of the century was the Dutchman Hermann Boerhaave, who like Sydenham upheld the Hippocratic doctrine of therapy depending on the curative powers of nature, and emphasized the importance of the doctor at the bedside. Instead of allowing his students to confine themselves to the theory of medicine, he also instructed them in bedside teaching.

father, a clergyman, wanted his son to follow in his footsteps and so Boerhaave studied theology and philosophy. He then turned to medicine, qualified, and in 1701 became professor of medicine and botany at the university of Leiden, which was the first to change the traditional methods of teaching.

As a doctor he was eclectic, accepting some concepts formulated by the iatrophysicists and the iatrochemists. His basic idea was pre-eminently Hippocratic and governed his teaching: the aim of medicine was to cure the sick and the doctor at the bedside must set aside all academic preconceptions and assess the situation calmly for himself. When a patient died, Boerhaave went with his pupils to the autopsy. To speak of his theories would be to detract from his greatness; it was for his teaching that he was most renowned and this was imparted at the courses held in the small hospital at Leiden. Every day with his students he went over the notes of each patient and then went on a round of visits, talking to patients and taking their temperatures.

His pupil the Swiss Albrecht von Haller (1708–77) had an astonishing output. He taught all branches of medicine, did an undefinable but certainly prodigious amount of work in anatomy and physiology, and created and directed botanical gardens. He also found time to write twelve books on physiology, four on anatomy, seven on botany, two on theology, four historical romances and limitless reviews in a scientific periodical at Göttingen, together with ten volumes of bibliography on botany, the medicinal properties of herbs, anatomy, surgery and medical practice, and he also wrote poetry. His great work *Elementa physiologiae corporis humani* (1757–66) marks the begining of the modern era, for the eight encyclopaedic volumes review the subject, discuss old concepts and present current views in the same way as a present-day work. Haller's most valuable contribution related to the physiology of the blood vessels and the nervous system.

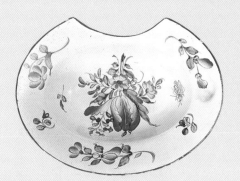

Above: a porcelain bleeding bowl, made in Strasbourg, circa 1760.

121...

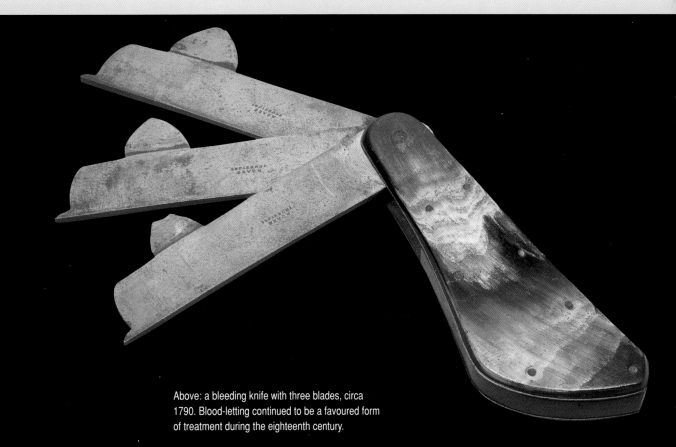

Above: a bleeding knife with three blades, circa 1790. Blood-letting continued to be a favoured form of treatment during the eighteenth century.

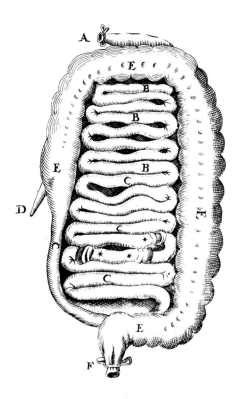

Above: the intestines as they were thought to be towards the end of the seventeenth century. An illustration from *Ephemeridum Medico-Physicarum Germanicorum*, c.1680.

...122

Galen had asserted that all sensibility was bound to the nervous system. Haller gave purely experimental definitions to irritability (which was present when contraction was observable) and sensibility (where stimulation was consciously noted – in man – or caused unrest – in animals) and showed by a long series of experiments that these two properties were distinct and independent, the former being a characteristic of muscle fibres and the latter of parts supplied by the nerves. Xavier Bichat (1771–1802) went on to state that these two phenomena were the basic characteristics of life. Haller is thus one of the founders of neurophysiology, but his studies embraced the anatomy, functions, and physical and chemical properties of all parts of the body as well as critical evaluation of all current experimental work.

Another pupil of Boerhaave's, the Dutchman Gerard van Swieten (1700–72), founded the old Viennese school. At that period the Austrian empire stretched westwards to Flanders and included a great part of northern Italy to the south. In 1744, the sister of the Empress Maria Theresa fell ill in Brussels and van Swieten was called in. The Empress was deeply impressed and invited him to become her personal doctor. The Dutchman was logically the successor to Boerhaave but he realised that as a Catholic his chances of obtaining the post in Protestant Leiden were small. He accepted the offer and went to Vienna, where, soon afterwards, he was given the job of reorganizing the faculty of medicine at the university.

Van Swieten separated the teaching of anatomy from that of surgery; he created a chemistry laboratory and an anatomy department and founded a botanical garden. Faithful to the system of his master Boerhaave, he had two wards at the hospital, one for male and one for female patients, reserved for the teaching of clinical medicine. The professors were no longer to be appointed by the faculty, but by the state, which paid their salaries and granted diplomas to those who studied medicine. Van Swieten was a celebrated clinician as well as a wise administrator with a long-term outlook. When he was still Boerhaave's assistant at Leiden, he wrote down the master's day-to-day comments on the cases, and he used this material in the compilation of five typically Hippocratic volumes entitled *Commentaria in Hermani Boerhaave aphorismos*.

The most distinguished doctor of the old Viennese school was Leopold Auenbrugger (1722–1809), who founded the science of physical diagnosis by developing percussion as a diagnostic method. The son of an innkeeper, he got the idea from the practice of tapping wine casks to find out how much they contained. He described the new technique of percussion in a little book, *Inventum novum*, published in 1761: by tapping lightly on the chest with the fingertips a note could be produced, the depth of which would indicate how much air was present in the thoracic cavity and whether or not the lungs were diseased. At first the discovery went almost unnoticed, but after Napoleon's doctor, Jean Nicolas Corvisart, translated Auenbrugger's work into French the new technique spread throughout the world.

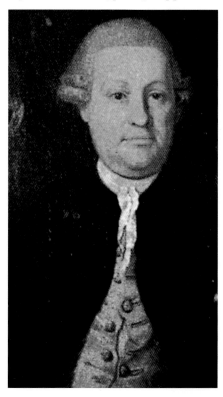

Right: Leopold Auenbrugger, who gave physical diagnosis the status of a science by his development of the method of percussion, interpreting the note produced by tapping the chest.

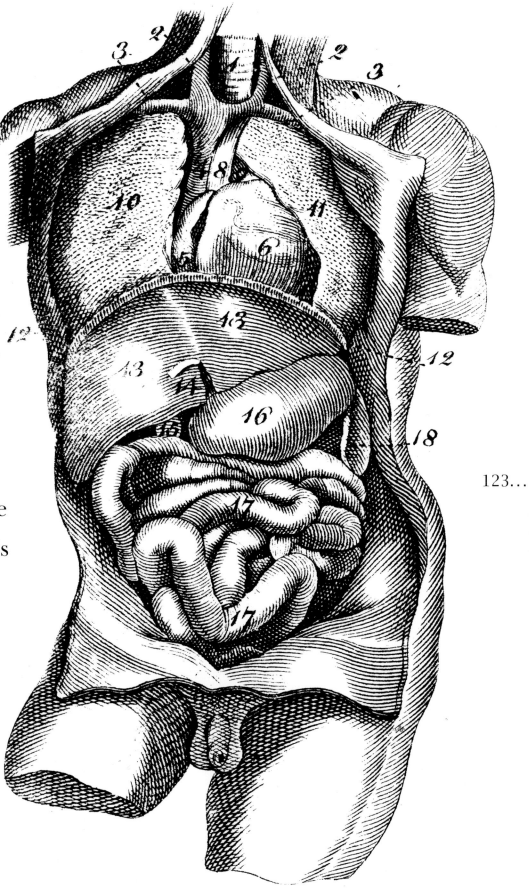

Gerard van Swieten established the first university clinic, while Leopold Auenbrugger founded the science of physical diagnosis by developing percussion as a diagnostic method.

123...

Above: the intestines as seen towards the end of the eighteenth century, showing considerable advances in anatomy over the illustration on the page opposite. A drawing from the first edition of the *Encyclopaedia Britannica*, 1768.

MORGAGNI, FOUNDER OF MODERN PATHOLOGY

In 1761, a work entitled *De sedibus et causis morborum* (On the sites and causes of diseases) was published in Italy. Its author was Giovanni Battista Morgagni (1682–1771), professor of anatomy at the university of Padua, and with it he laid the foundations of pathological anatomy. Morgagni studied the anatomical difference between the unhealthy and the healthy body, linking symptoms to abnormalities in the body.

Morgagni's discoveries were legion. He made classic descriptions, to name only a few conditions, of angina pectoris, myocardial degeneration, and subacute bacterial endocarditis, and distinguished postmortem blood clots in the chambers of the heart from vegetations formed in life. He also made original observations on tuberculosis of the lungs and described vividly a tubercle in the process of liquefaction. His work on tumours of the pylorus is noteworthy. He showed that urethral discharge (as in gonorrhoea) occurs independently of penile ulcers (as in syphilis).

Morgagni stated that strokes did not come primarily from a lesion of the brain but rather from changes in the cerebral blood vessels. He was the first to connect syphilis with disease of the cerebral arteries and he noted that hemiplegia affected the side of the body opposite that of the cerebral hemisphere which had been damaged, and that hemiplegia did not result from lesions of the cerebellum. It should be borne in mind that crossed hemiplegia had been noted in Smith's papyrus and in Hippocrates's *On cranial fractures*; the pyramidal decussation had been anatomically described by Mestichelli of Rome in 1710. There is no aspect of pathological anatomy in which Morgagni did not excel. More than two centuries after his death his work remains alive and complete, so that one can today give exact diagnosis to the cases that he describes.

...124

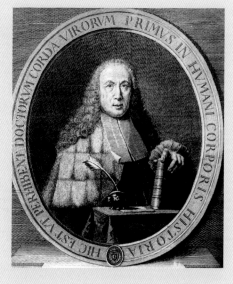

Above: Giovanni Battista Morgagni, a tireless investigator and for fifty-six years professor of anatomy at the university of Padua.

Right: Antoine-Laurent Lavoisier, who completed the theory of respiration, with his wife, 1788, by Jacques Louis David.

Morgagni had many distinguished students, among them Lazzaro Spallanzani (1729–99), who carried out remarkable biological work and made fundamentally important contributions to the study of the digestion, circulation, regeneration and reproduction. The concept of spontaneous generation, that is of the birth of animals from decomposing matter, was still actively discussed but Spallanzani showed, in the case of the frog, that spermatozoa from the male were needed for fertilization of the female ova.

Harvey had written that all living beings share in common an origin either from the seed or the egg, leaving the question of whether the seed or egg derived from beings of the same species unanswered. Spallanzani demonstrated that the frog, placed on the back of the female, showered the eggs with sperm as they were produced. He then showed that the fertilizing power of the male fluid was suppressed if its direct contact with the eggs was prevented by covering the male parts with waxed cloth, but that the male fluid so obtained, when placed in contact with the eggs, fertilized them.

Spallanzani used a method devised by Rene de Reaumur (1683–1757), inventor of a scale for thermometers and of the alcohol thermometer. Reaumur prepared metal tubes closed at either end by a fine metal mesh and, having filled them with food, he made kites ingest them; these birds regurgitate what they have not digested. Spallanzani experimented similarly with birds and

> **Morgagni is regarded as the founder of scientific pathological anatomy – the study of the appearance of the body in disease.**

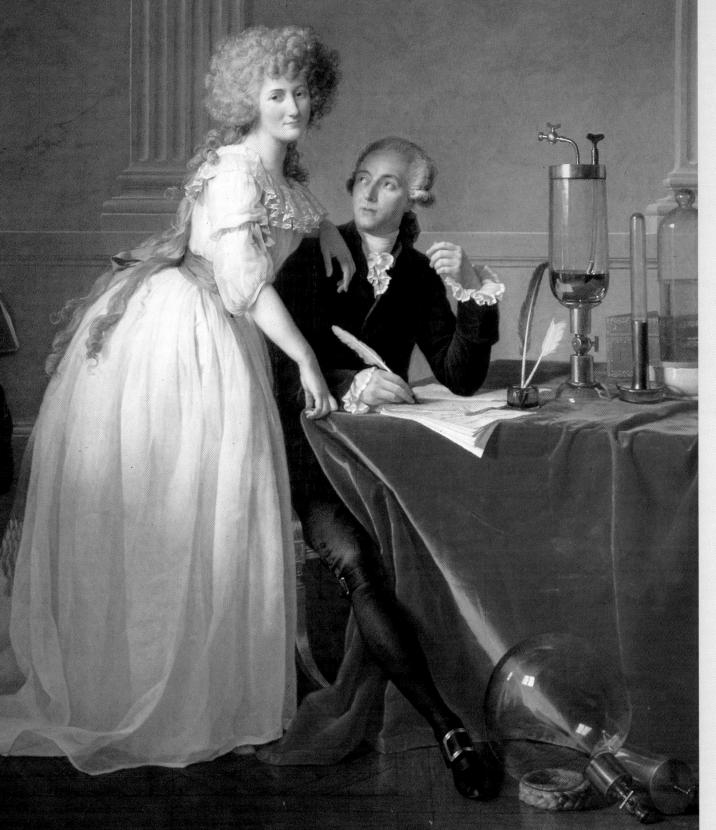

confirmed Reaumur's findings that digestion was not a process of trituration and putrefaction of food, as was then believed, and went on to show that gastric juice dissolved food. Spallanzani, making use of Lavoisier's discoveries, increased knowledge of the physiology of respiration, and showed that asphyxiated animals died from brain damage due to lack of oxygen.

Antoine-Laurent Lavoisier(1743–94) was both the father of modern chemistry and an eminent physiologist. He showed that respiration was a process of combustion, with the utilization of the oxygen and the production of carbon dioxide, and applied his discovery to public health, demonstrating the need for a certain quantity of air per head in confined inhabited spaces.

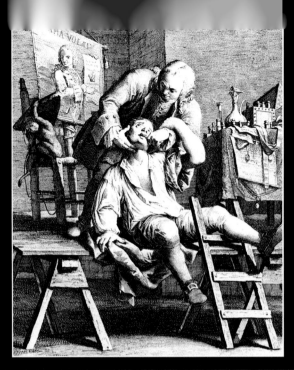

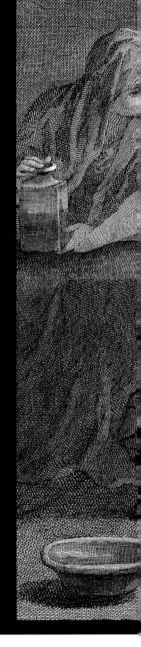

Lavoisier's work was the culmination of extensive studies on the physiology of respiration carried out during the eighteenth century in several countries, notably in England. The different gases of the atmosphere had been discovered: carbon dioxide by Joseph Black (1728–99) in 1757, hydrogen by Henry Cavendish (1731–1810) in 1766, nitrogen by Daniel Rutherford (1749–1819) in 1772. Joseph Priestley (1733–1804) had isolated oxygen in 1772, but was confused by Stahl's theory, whereby substances were supposed on burning (oxidation) to lose something called phlogiston – even though an increase in weight was observed; Priestley called oxygen 'dephlogisticated air'. It was Lavoisier who finally discovered the true nature of the process by which oxygen is taken up by the blood in the lungs.

Special study began at this time on the electrical phenomena of muscles and nerves. When muscles contract, energy, heat and electrical activity are generated. When the nervous impulse passes along a nerve it is manifested by an electrical phenomenon, the action potential. The electrical changes in these tissues can be detected in various ways, both directly and in other parts of the body. The investigation of animal electricity began with the experiments of Luigi Galvani (1737–98) and Alessandro Volta (1745–1827). Using a skinned frog, Galvani observed that by touching the nerves or the muscles with a piece of metal connected to an electrostatic machine, the muscles could be made to contract. The interpretation of this phenomenon was the cause of a lengthy difference of opinion between Galvani and Volta, who repeated the experiments and became convinced that electricity was not inherent in the organism but was due to the contact of the different metals of the conducting circuit.

Volta developed his concept and invented the battery; electric current was thus produced for the first time. Electrophysiology advanced some years later when, in 1841, the Italian physiologist Carlo Matteucci (1811–68) showed that all muscular activity was accompanied by an electrical phenomenon. He placed the sciatic nerve of a frog in contact with muscle fibres of another frog. By stimulating the nerve of the second frog, Matteucci produced a secondary contraction in the muscles of the first. These experiments laid the foundation of neurophysiology and electroencephalography, while they were applied in practice in electrotherapy, with benefit in some neuromuscular disorders.

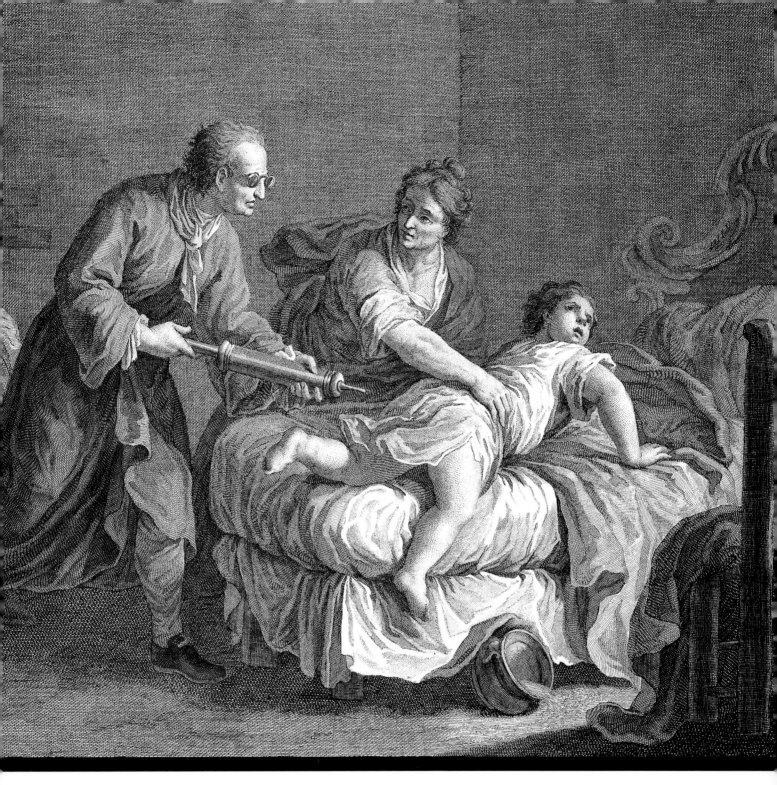

Lavoisier demonstrated that respiration was a process of combustion, burning up the oxygen in the air and producing carbon dioxide. He applied his discovery to public health, showing the need for a given amount of air per head in confined spaces.

MESMERISM AND HOMEOPATHY

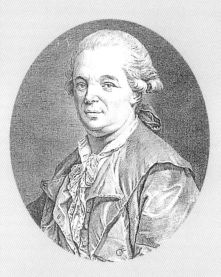

Franz Anton Mesmer (1734–1815) qualified in medicine at Vienna with a thesis entitled *De planetarum influxu*, which showed how the planets exercised an influence on the tissues of the human body both in health and disease. He attributed this to a mysterious fluid which he later named 'animal magnetism'. He introduced magnetic therapy, which derived from the laying of hands on the sick patient, a method which he claimed to have produced remarkable cures. He straddled the worlds of orthodox and dubious medicine.

Mesmer was born in a village on Lake Constance. After qualifying in Vienna, he settled there and married a wealthy young widow and moved in fashionable circles. Early in 1763 he became a controversial figure when the sight of a girl was partly restored by his methods; the girl, Maria Paradies, had been blind since the age of three and a half. Doctors in Vienna started intriguing against him and he moved to Paris where he soon became one of the most popular physicians on account of his power of healing the sick and ending pain by inducing a state of trance. Mesmer earned enormous sums of money and enjoyed the patronage of Queen Marie Antoinette. Louis XVI offered him an income of 20,000 francs to remain in Paris and an additional 10,000 francs if he opened a Magnetic Institute there. But a dispute with established French physicians forced Mesmer to forgo the king's attractive offer and he retired to Spa. However his numerous admirers formed an association in his support, collected 340,000 francs and agitated loudly for his return.

Above: Mesmer, whose treatments using 'animal magnetism' drew crowds of the rich and famous.

...128

Mesmer's fame was such that his clients included famous writers, aristocrats, generals and politicians, and appointments had to be made weeks in advance. Clients were ushered into magnificent consulting rooms where they found others around a bath of dilute sulphuric acid from which curved iron bars protruded. The lights would dim, perfume would fill the air and distant music would create a suitable atmosphere. The patients grasped the bars or joined hands and formed a circle. Then Mesmer would appear in a scarlet silk robe and touch each patient in turn in different places, inducing a hypnotic trance during which he would suggest that they were cured. On returning home, his visitors would be convinced that they were better.

A commission was set up with four members of the Academy of Medicine and five from the Academy of Sciences, including Benjamin Franklin and Lavoisier. They conducted an enquiry into Mesmer's system of treatment and gave an unfavourable verdict. 'Nothing proves the existence of magnetic animal fluid; imagination without magnetism may produce convulsions; magnetism without imagination produces nothing.' Despite official disapproval, Mesmer could not be accused of chicanery for he acted in all good faith. On the other hand, his enthusiastic admirers sincerely believed in animal magnetism. and Mesmer certainly proved the power of the imagination.

One of Mesmer's pupils observed that the greatest benefit occurred in the case of patients who were unconscious of any other stimulus during the sessions, and concentrated all their attention on the magnetizer, accepting without question everything that Mesmer suggested to them. When they came round these patients remembered nothing whatsoever of what had taken place. This is characteristic of the state produced by hypnosis, the most important aspect of Mesmer therapy.

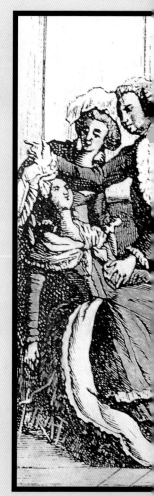

In Mesmer's wake came many quacks and adventurers who earned a great deal of money by playing on the gullibility of others. One of the best known was Guiseppe Balsamo (1743–95) known as Count Alessandro di Cagliostro. A doctor and occultist to whom miraculous cures were ascribed, he was a fashionable physician at Louis XVI's court in Mesmer's time. He was involved in a scandal with the Cardinal de Rohan and Countess de la Motte, a lady of fortune, and fled to Rome. Later he was imprisoned as a heretic, freemason and swindler. Another was Dr James Graham (1745–94) of Edinburgh. Graham had studied some medicine and picked up something of Benjamin Franklin's experiments with electricity in the United States. In London, he first set up 'celestial beds' for restoring virility and fertility, then a 'temple of health' (admission six guineas) and, when this fraud was exposed, a mudbath establishment.

It is at this period that the system of homeopathy emerged. Homeopathic therapy consists essentially in the use, at minimal dosage levels, of substances which in a greater dose provoked symptoms similar to those of the disease they were supposed to cure. The founder of this form of treatment was the German Samuel Friedrich Hahnemann (1755–1843), who upheld the principle '*similia similibus curantur*' (like is cured by like), after having experimented on himself with various medicines. Thus hot compresses were used for burns and opium for inducing sleep.

Below: a coloured engraving satirizing Mesmer's treatment, circa 1783.

129...

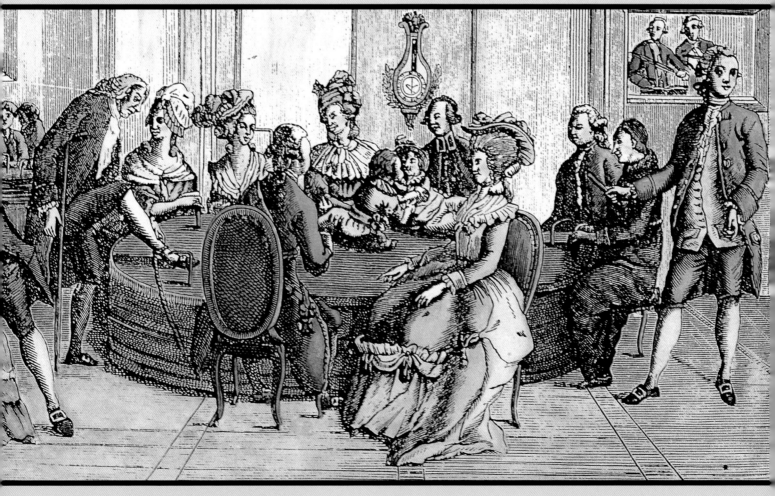

JENNER AND THE DISCOVERY OF VACCINATION

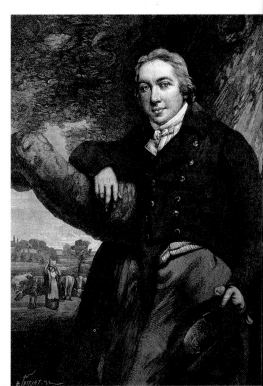

Edward Jenner (1749–1823), who was born in Berkeley in Gloucestershire, is among the most admirable and likeable figures in the history of medicine. From his boyhood he was determined to become a doctor and at the age of thirteen he became a surgeon's assistant near Bristol, where he remained for six years. One day a young country girl came to the surgery and the conversation turned to the subject of smallpox; she said: 'I cannot take that disease, for I have had cowpox'. This phrase impressed itself on Jenner who observed its truth among farmers and their families. When he was twenty-one he went to London, where he became the pupil and friend of the celebrated Scots surgeon John Hunter (1728–93), founder of pathological anatomy in England.

A former naval surgeon, John Hunter was not an academic but a fervid and intelligent experimenter, who became the victim of one of his own experi-

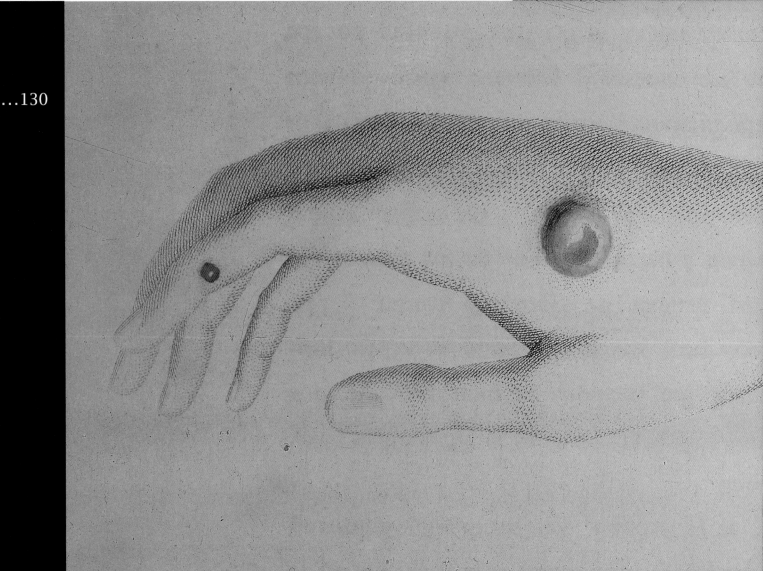

ments. In an attempt to find out if gonorrhoea and syphilis were two different diseases or merely two forms of the same disease, he inoculated himself with pus from a patient. As luck would have it, he had chosen a patient infected with both conditions. This circumstance led him to state, erroneously, that gonorrhoea and syphilis were one and the same; and it also produced a syphilitic aortic aneurysm, which killed him.

Hunter's elder brother William (1718–1873) was the most noted British anatomist of the eighteenth century and author of a great and monumental work, *The Anatomy of the Gravid Uterus*, published by the famous Birmingham printer John Baskerville; the work contained 34 copper plates that were masterpieces of anatomical illustration.

After two years, Jenner returned to Berkeley to be a country doctor. In Gloucestershire, it had long been common knowledge that dairy maids who caught cowpox were immune to smallpox. This must have been known the length and breadth of England, for smallpox had been widespread for at least two hundred years. Although its origins in Britain are obscure, smallpox gradually became more common but did not reach epidemic importance until the reign of James I. In his *History of Epidemics in Britain* (1894), Creighton wrote: 'It first left the richer classes, then it left the villages, then it left the provincial

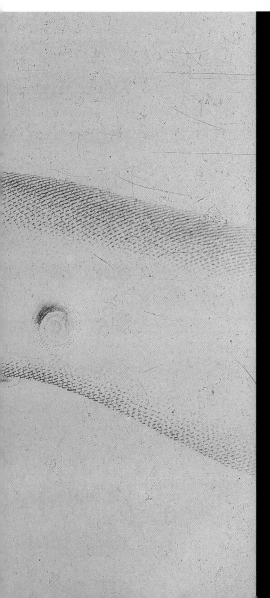

A new era of preventative medicine began in 1796, when Edward Jenner pioneered the use of the cowpox vaccine to produce immunity to smallpox. The practice was at once widely adopted, soon controlling a disease which had previously been one of mankind's greatest plagues.

131...

Top: Edward Jenner, the country doctor, in his native Gloucestershire.

Left: a coloured engraving showing the hand of the dairy maid, Sarah Nelmes, with the cowpox pustules from which Jenner made his smallpox vaccine in 1796.

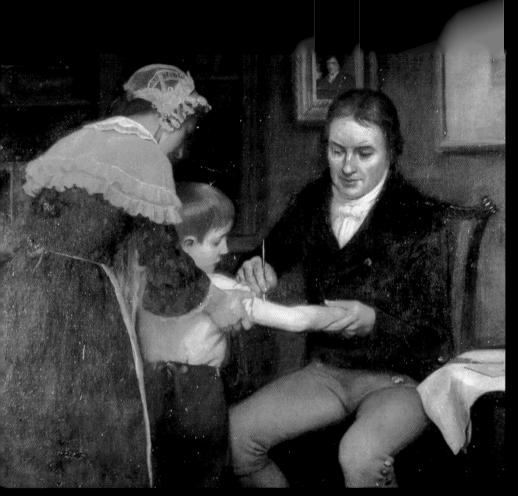

Left: Edward Jenner vaccinating James Phipps with lymph taken from the cowpox pustules on Sarah Nelmes's hand. 14 May 1796. A painting by Ernest Board, circa 1915.

Below: a contemporary cartoon suggesting the possible effects of the smallpox vaccination. In spite of its obvious effectiveness and safety, the smallpox vaccination was a target for ill-informed and superstitious criticism for a long time.

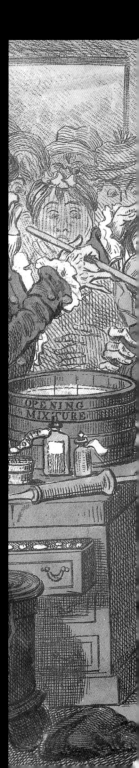

towns to centre itself in the capital; at the same time it was leaving the age of infancy and childhood.' It has been calculated that smallpox claimed a total of 60,000,000 lives in eighteenth-century Europe.

Variolation or variolization was known in England from 1717, when Lady Mary Wortley Montagu, the wife of the English ambassador in Constantinople, who had seen it practised among the Turks, described it in detail in a letter to a friend. Variolation was carried out by inoculating material from persons suffering from mild varieties of smallpox, in order to reproduce the benign form of the disease and thus prevent more serious forms from developing. Although this procedure provided a defence it was also very risky, sometimes producing a serious infection even when the primary disease was ostensibly benign.

Given that smallpox was a variable disease, inoculation of infected material offered the possibility of preventing treatment. Jenner studied the problem systematically; it took him twenty years to complete his work with a decisive experiment. This was carried out on 14 May 1796, when he extracted the contents of pustule on the hand of a milkmaid affected by cowpox and inoculated it into the arm of a healthy eight-year-old boy. This had no ill effects, and the experiment was a success, for six weeks later Jenner inoculated the child with material from human smallpox pustules and the boy did not catch smallpox. Jenner repeated the experiment on others; when he was quite certain that he had made a valid discovery, he referred the matter to the Royal Society, of which he had been made a fellow for his zoological work. His report was returned to him with a note explaining that he would do best not to endanger the reputation he had gained for his previous studies by continuing with his present work. But Jenner was confident of his observations and did not take the well-meant advice. His study was published in 1798 under the title *An Inquiry*

The treatise aroused violent emotions, but all that mattered was that smallpox vaccination became known and practised everywhere within as short a space of time possible. Jenner gained just recognition, and in 1802 Parliament voted him a grant of £10,000 and in 1808 he was appointed by the government as director for its newly-formed institute for vaccination. His discovery resulted from masterful experience and observation, although Jenner himself was constantly saddened by his inability to explain why his system worked. It was another hundred years before the basic features of immunity were revealed, but Jenner's genius and perseverance nevertheless produced in his time an empirical triumph of preventive medicine.

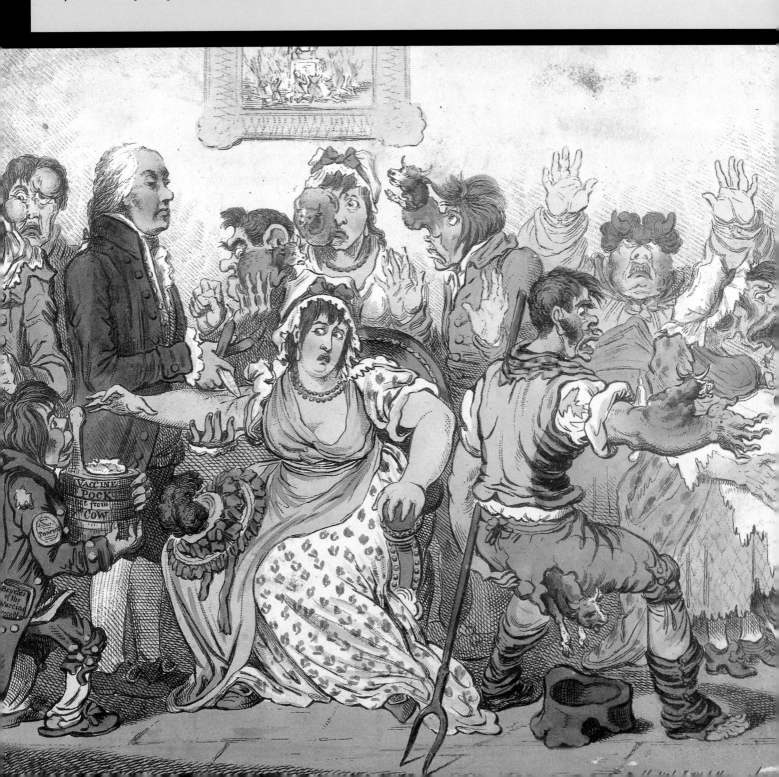

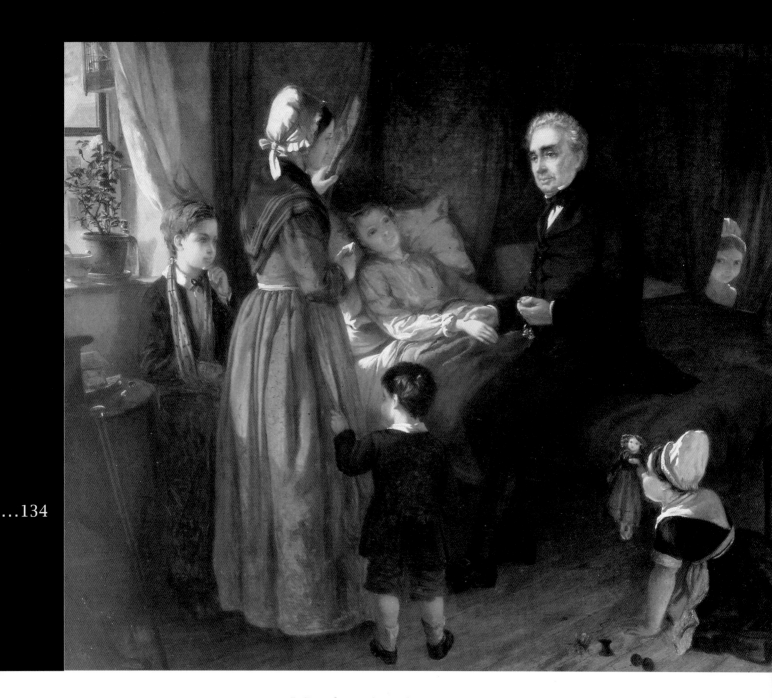

Mechanization and industrial development in the early nineteenth century benefited medicine directly through the invention of new diagnostic and therapeutic instruments, among them Laënnec's stethoscope, Helmholtz's opthalmoscope, for examining the interior of the eye, and the hypodermic syringe.

THE ERA OF
GREAT CONQUESTS

The nineteenth century was a period of rapidly accelerating change, and the spirit of scientific thought and enquiry pervaded all branches of knowledge. The universities began to break free of ecclesiastical and political control, and study there became possible for members of social classes formerly excluded. The great English naturalist Charles Darwin (1809–82) gave the theory of evolution a scientific foundation by correlating masses of biological data within the framework of a single idea; in his work *On the origin of species* (1859), he expounded the law of natural selection, which opened new horizons in medicine. Of vital importance, too, were the discovery in 1845 of the law of the conservation of energy by Robert Jules Mayer and by James Prescott Joule, and of a fundamental law of genetics by Gregor Mendel (1822–84).

Mechanization and industrial development in the early nineteenth century benefited medicine directly through the invention of new diagnostic and therapeutic instruments. One of the earliest of these was Laënnec's stethoscope (page 140); others of great importance were Helmholtz's ophthalmoscope and the hypodermic syringe introduced in 1853 by the Frenchman Charles Pravaz and Alexander Wood of Edinburgh.

The first years of the nineteenth century saw the development of modern chemistry and particularly biochemistry. Much of the important work in the field was carried out in Germany, which retained its lead for many years. An epoch-making event was the laboratory production of urea from an inorganic substance, ammonium carbonate, by the German Friedrich Wöhler (1800–82) in 1828. Before Wöhler's synthesis it was believed that organic compounds, the chemicals of life, could be formed only by living tissue and were totally distinct from mineral or inorganic substances. Following the work of the English chemist John Dalton, Justus von Liebig (1803–73) investigated many organic chemical compounds, both in and derived from food and in waste products, and discovered among many other things chloral and chloroform.

The Industrial Revolution created a new society, with rural populations moving to the towns. Cities developed so fast that public health suffered; slums grew rapidly, with unhealthy and overcrowded dwellings. Lavoisier (pages 125–6) had found that in a closed environment the air soon deteriorated as the oxygen was used up, and he urged the need for living space to be made the subject of legislation. But this was a liberal era – 'laissez faire, laissez passer' – and no controls were imposed, even over water and food.

The new United States of America was ready to contribute to all fields of knowledge, but especially to medicine. Its first medical school had been founded in 1765 at Philadelphia by John Morgan (1735–89), on the best European models. Morgan worked in London with the Hunter brothers, qualified at Edinburgh, lived in Paris and travelled through Italy where he made the acquaintance of Morgagni.

The most popular doctor of the War of Independence was Benjamin Rush (1745–1813) 'the American Sydenham', a product of the Philadelphia school. He was well known in Europe for his work on yellow fever, the vector of which he believed to be the mosquito, and as a pioneer in physiotherapy. He wrote an important psychiatric work, but at the time of Pinel's reforms he advocated the use of a barbarous 'tranquillizing chair'.

135...

Above: in The Sickroom by Emma Brownlow (fl.1852–77), an old family doctor sits at the bedside of a young female patient.

Ephraim McDowell (1771–1830) is remembered as one of the first to remove diseased ovaries. His first patient, Mrs Crawford of Danville, Kentucky, was operated on under primitive conditions in a remote country village, without antiseptics or anaesthesia. She sang hymns while he removed her tumour, with a crowd waiting anxiously outside the house. McDowell enjoyed phenomenal success at the time and achieved international fame when eight of his thirteen patients were cured.

The most internationally famous American doctor was William Beaumont (1785–1853). His career developed in a unique way from that of frontier surgeon to physiologist specializing in the mechanism of digestion. In 1812 he became camp surgeon at Fort Mackinac, a trading post on Lake Erie, and the incident marking the turning point in his career took place there in 1822. Alexis Saint Martin, a nineteen-year-old trapper, was accidently shot in the stomach. Beaumont dressed the severe wound but felt that Saint Martin had only a few hours to live. But he survived the wound and a difficult opera-

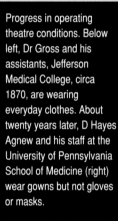

Progress in operating theatre conditions. Below left, Dr Gross and his assistants, Jefferson Medical College, circa 1870, are wearing everyday clothes. About twenty years later, D Hayes Agnew and his staff at the University of Pennsylvania School of Medicine (right) wear gowns but not gloves or masks.

...136

Until the nineteenth century, medicine had progressed by fits and starts, but now developments came quickly and specialization appeared for the first time.

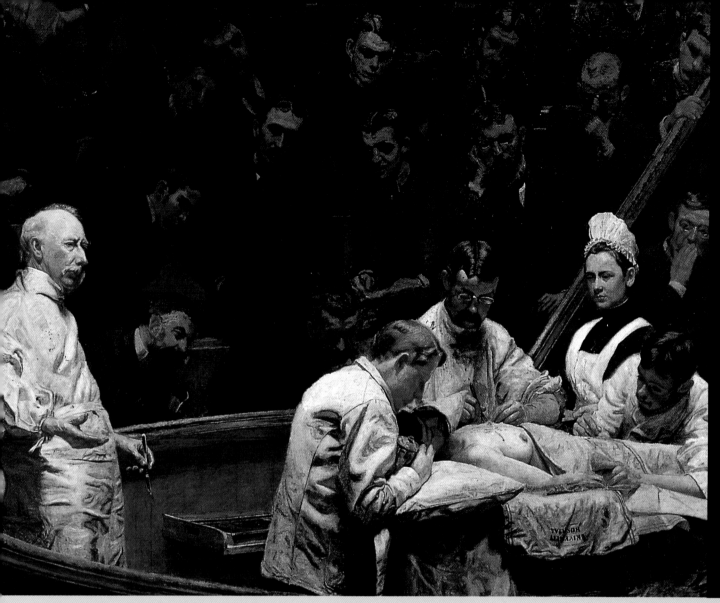

tion was carried out successfully. In two years, under Beaumont's care, Alexis had recovered, but with a permanent gastric fistula. Beaumont was able to see directly into the cavity of the young man's stomach, and he began to study the digestive process at work. Although without academic training, his research was impeccably methodical and successfully provided accurate information, which led to the formation of theories that are still valid.

In fact the American surgeon studied the whole field of gastric physiology, observing carefully the contractions of the stomach and various changes in its lining in different phases of digestion. He investigated the manifestations of hunger and thirst. He described the appearance and properties of gastric juice and determined the presence of hydrochloric acid and other active substances in the stomach. He found that the stomach was a contractile sac, separated from the duodenum by the pylorus, which periodically opened like a valve to allow food digested by the gastric juices to pass onwards. Peristaltic contractions had two functions, to mix the food with gastric secretions and to enable the stomach to empty the products of digestion.

In the nineteenth century, medicine developed rapidly in Europe and America. Until then progress in medicine had been episodic, with triumphs and fresh concepts alternating with long periods of stagnation. Now, new developments came so quickly that knowledge of all aspects of medical science became impossible for individuals to attain, and specialization appeared for the first time. Medical knowledge, now embracing huge and diverse fields, split into several distinct branches.

THE SCHOOL OF PARIS

It could be said that Napoleon was an important and permanent influence on medicine; undoubtedly he encouraged the work of a number of great clinicians and scientists in the first years of the nineteenth century and so laid the foundations of a great school. The first giant of this Parisian school was Marie François Xavier Bichat (1771–1802), who carried out work of fundamental importance in his short life. In his *Anatomie generale*, Bichat showed that all organs were made up of a smaller number of tissues, which he described both in the healthy and diseased state. In the masterly *Recherches physiologiques sur la vie et la mort*, Bichat distinguished two types of functions, those of vegetative and those of animal life. Through the latter, higher organisms were able to perceive the external world, respond to stimuli, move and display desires and emotions. Through the vegetative functions, that is the circulation of the blood, respiration, digestion, metabolism and temperature regulation, they took in and utilized materials from outside (food, water, air) and then excreted the waste products. Bichat had a strong influence on the most celebrated clinician of the First Empire, Jean Nicolas Corvisart (1755–1821), Napoleon's personal physician, who translated Auenbrugger's book on percussion and so led to the general adoption of the technique. He was a cardiologist, defining symptoms due to heart diseases and distinguishing them from the pulmonary symptoms. It is said that one day he studied a portrait and remarked: 'If the painter was right, the man in this picture died of heart disease'. This was shown to be so.

Another favourite of Napoleon was Jean Dominique Larrey (1766–1842), the chief doctor of the Grande Armée. Larrey was the first to institute field units to give first aid and immediate surgery to the wounded, and experimented with refrigeration to dull the pain of amputation. In November 1812, when Napoleon's troops were fighting the Russian army under Kutosov, he performed more than two hundred amputations within the space of twenty-four hours and without getting any sleep. The emperor left him a legacy of 100,000 francs and made him a baron.

Napoleon also conferred baronies on Corvisart and on Guillaume Dupuytren (1777–1835), the chief surgeon at the Hôtel-Dieu. Dupuytren left classic descriptions of the characteristic flexion of fingers caused by contraction of ligamentous tissue in the palm (Dupuytren's contraction) and of fracture of the lower end of the fibula (Dupuytren's fracture).

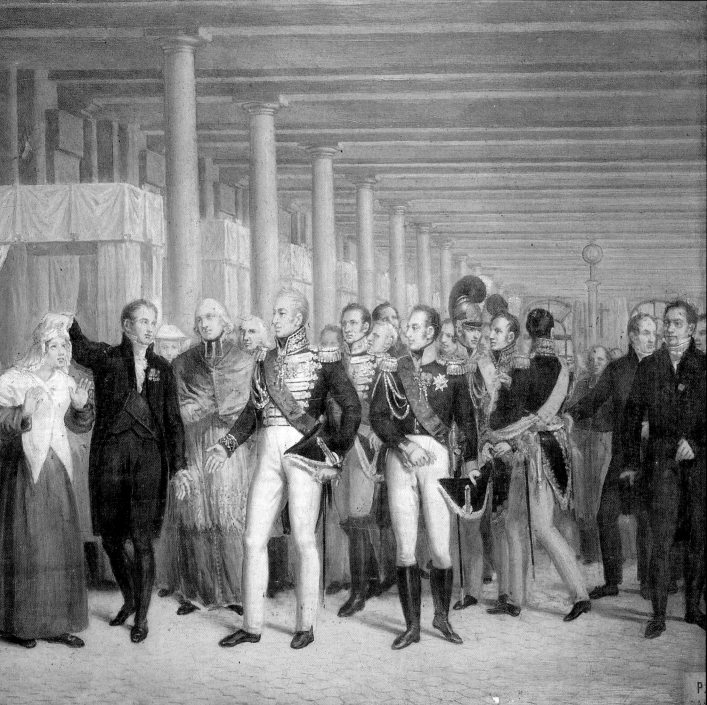

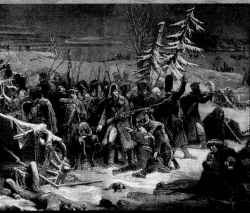

Top: following a successful operation to remove a cataract at the Hôtel-Dieu, Dupuytren presents his patient to Charles X.

Above: the retreat from Moscow, 1812. Only one thousand of the Grande Armée were fit for action when the French withdrew from Russian territory.

When Napoleon dominated Europe politically, doctors of the Paris school played a leading role in medicine. Bichat was a pioneer of pathology, Larrey the greatest of military surgeons, and Dupuytren another leading surgeon, whose name lives on in Dupuytren's contraction and Dupuytren's fracture.

Right: Laënnec's original stethoscope of 1819. It is a wooden tube about 23 cm (9 in) long and 4 cm (1½ in) in diameter, consisting of two parts which screw into one another and a detachable chest-piece.

Corvisart's greatest pupil was René Theophile Hyacinthe Laënnec (1781–1826), the inventor of the stethoscope and the first man to create a complete diagnostic system for pulmonary and cardiac complaints. For many years Laënnec was obsessed with a desire to hear clearly the noises of opening and closure of the heart valves in systole and diastole, to achieve accurate diagnosis. It is said that one day, while crossing the courtyard of the Louvre, he saw a boy listening with his ear at the end of a wooden beam to signals tapped by another child with a nail on the other end. At the first opportunity during the examination of a patient, Laënnec put a roll of paper to his chest and found that he heard the heart sounds more clearly, and even better when he replaced the roll of paper with a cylinder of turned wood, to which he gave the name stethoscope. Thomas Addison commented that Laënnec's writings contributed more toward the advance of medicine than the work of any other single individual.

...140

Pierre Louis (1787–1872) is remembered today as the man who introduced statistical methods into medicine, and in the 'angle of Louis', the prominence in the upper part of the breastbone. As a young man he spent six years in Russia and became disillusioned by the powerlessness of medicine to cope with severe epidemic infections. He returned to Paris to study and spent the rest of his life in hospitals, researching and teaching. In the course of his work he became convinced that fallacious theories or arguments could be refuted by a careful statistical analysis of the medical evidence, and that statistics could be used to give a convincing result on occasions where experiments could not be carried out. His work has proved of lasting value: Louis's methods have been used to determine the effectiveness or otherwise of new treatments for particular diseases. His chief works were his *Recherches anatomico-physiologiques sur la phthisie* (1825), which was based on nearly 2,000 cases and showed the frequent occurrence of tuberculosis in the apex of the lung, and his *Recherches* on typhoid fever (1829) which gave the disease its present name.

In Magendie's words, 'The aim of science is to substitute facts for appearances and demonstrations for impressions.'

The physiologist Joseph François Magendie (1783–1855) made a number of important discoveries, which however he never attempted to synthesize. He affirmed the necessity of obtaining knowledge from animal experiments. 'The aim of science', he said, 'is to substitute facts for appearances and demonstrations for impressions.' Today he is remembered for his discovery of the sensory function of the posterior roots of spinal nerves. But he was also the founder of modern pharmacology; by demonstrating the action on animals of such substances as strychnine and morphine he gave a scientific basis for the clinical use of these drugs. In fact modern therapy had begun some years earlier with the publication (1786) by William Withering on the effectiveness of digitalis in cer-

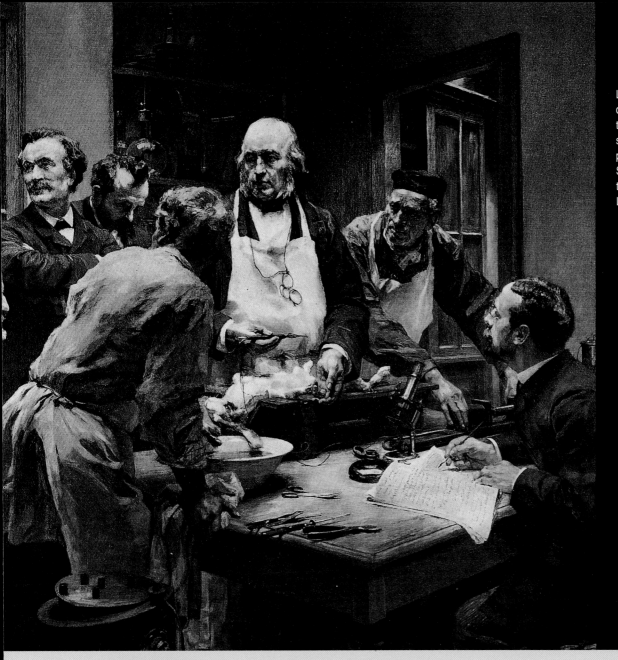

Left: Claude Bernard dissecting a rabbit, in the company of several noted professors at the Sorbonne, 1899. After the painting by L L'hermitte.

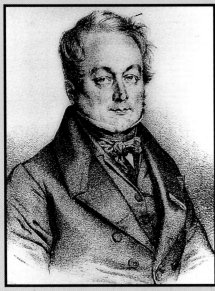

Above: François Magendie, who emphasized the importance of an experimental basis for research; he is said to have refused to believe any statement that had not been confirmed.

tain heart conditions. Soon afterwards, the pharmacopoeia of the Royal College of Physicians in London finally discarded the archaic remedies that included animal organs and excreta, while during the early nineteenth century quinine, atropine, morphine and strychnine were isolated.

Magendie's favourite pupil was Claude Bernard (1813–78) whose achievements embraced every branch of physiology; with the imagination of genius he was able to synthesize the findings from his experiments into fundamental doctrines.

After a false start as a pharmacist, he turned to playwriting and went to Paris with a letter of introduction to a celebrated critic. The critic, Saint-Marc Girardin, a professor at the Sorbonne, read Bernard's play and said: 'My dear boy, you have been working in a pharmacy and your head is full of ideas. It is science you want, not the theatre.'

Bernard then enrolled in the faculty of medicine, and, when he qualified, became Magendie's assistant at the Collège de France. His lectures were published in several volumes between 1854 and 1878, the year of his death. One of his first discoveries was based on his observation that sugar was found in the blood coming from the liver of a dog whether the animal was fed meat or sugar, thus the liver had a glycogenic (sugar-forming) function. Bernard initiated modern metabolic studies by showing the synthesis and breakdown of a substance (glycogen) in the body.

Above: ganglion under the jaw of a calf. One of Claude Bernard's watercolours based on his dissections, now in the archives of the Collège de France.

Equally important was his work on vasomotor nerves which constrict and dilate blood vessels and so control the flow of blood under varying conditions to different parts of the body. By cutting the sympathetic nerves he showed that they cause constriction, while the parasympathetic nerves were necessary for glandular secretion as they increased blood flow. By producing a pancreatic fistula he discovered that pancreatic juice was important for digestion (previously thought to occur only in the stomach), breaking down fats, starch and protein. But perhaps his greatest achievement was his *Leçons sur les phenomenes de la vie* (1878), in which he stated his doctrine of the constancy of the 'internal environment'. This concept was neglected for many years, but with the growth of knowledge of interdependent hormones and the equilibria of many bodily processes (homeostasis) it is now accepted as one of the fundamental principles of physiology.

Bernard's successor at the Collège de France was Charles Edouard Brown-Séquard (1817–94), born on the island of Mauritius of an American sea captain father and a French mother. He studied medicine in Paris and travelled a great deal in the USA and England, teaching at Harvard and practising at the National Hospital, Queen Square, London, returning to Paris after Bernard's death in 1878. Claude Bernard wrote: 'It may be held that the total internal secretions constitute the blood which should thus, in my opinion, be held to be a true product of internal secretion', thus anticipating the discovery of hormones, the blood-borne secretions of the endocrine glands. Brown-Séquard took note of Addison's observations on the effects of disease of the adrenals and by experiment proved that these glands were essential to life, and was thus a pioneer of endocrinology.

Since his time, two hormones have been found to be produced by the adrenal medulla: adrenaline (isolated in 1901 by Takamine and synthesized in 1904 by Stolz) and noradrenaline. The former produces constriction of the skin and digestive blood vessels and relaxation of visceral muscles, while the latter is the true mediator of sympathetic nerve impulses. After Jacques Loeb (1859–1924) showed the important function of the cortical (outer) zone of the adrenal glands, E C Kendall (1886–1972) and his colleagues succeeded in 1936 in isolating various cortical steroid hormones. In the same year T Reichstein (b. 1897) also discovered a number of corticosteroids, among them cortisone, which has found many applications in the treatment of inflammatory and some malignant conditions as well as in Addison's disease.

The term hormone was used for the first time in 1902 by the British W M Bayliss (1860–1924) and E H Starling (1866–1927), who discovered secretin, a substance produced by the duodenal mucous membrane and passed directly into the blood, thus determining the secretion of pancreatic juice without the

Claude's crowning achievement was his concept of the body's 'internal environment', which is kept constant by several interacting, self-regulating mechanisms. The nervous system is one, hormones another.

143...

intervention of the nervous system. Insulin, the active principle of the islets of Langerhans in the pancreas, which regulates sugar metabolism, was isolated in 1921. Merit of discovery belongs to the Canadian Frederick G Banting (1891–1941), who in 1923 won a Nobel prize, and to Charles Best (1899–1978). Insulin came into therapeutic use straightaway as a treatment for diabetes, where the body is unable to use sugar as a food.

Repeated mention of Thomas Addison (1795–1860) should prompt us to consider briefly what might be called the Guy's school, which flourished in London in the middle of the nineteenth century. The three great men of Guy's Hospital were Addison, Richard Bright (1798–1858) and Thomas Hodgkin (1798–1866), and each is remembered with an eponymous disease.

Addison produced early accounts of appendicitis and toxicology. His essay, published in 1855, *On the Constitutional and Local Effects of Disease of the Suprarenal Capsules*, contained descriptions of both Addison's disease and pernicious anaemia, but the significance of his observations remained largely unrecognized during his lifetime.

Richard Bright, whose name is attached to glomerulonephritis, was an Edinburgh graduate like Addison. He travelled in Iceland and Hungary, as artist, naturalist and geographer, and left lucid descriptions of many diseases. He established at Guy's in 1842 what may have been the first clinical research unit, with two wards for kidney patients with a laboratory and consulting room attached. The third great name, Hodgkin, was a pathologist rather than a clinician. His skill is attested by re-examination of his specimens of Hodgkin's disease – enlargement of lymph nodes and lymphatic tissue – which survive to this day. The microscope, which he did not use, confirms his diagnosis.

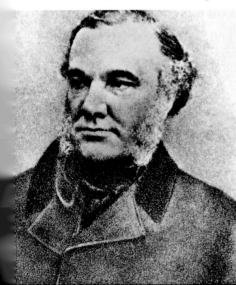

Above: Thomas Addison of Guy's Hospital, London, who made outstanding contributions to the studies of pernicious anaemia and chronic disease of the adrenal glands.

ANAESTHESIA

Although surgery had progressed since the Middle Ages when it was seen as a skilled manual craft unworthy of the attention of the medical profession proper, nevertheless, at the beginning of the nineteenth century it had limited horizons. The solution of four difficult problems – pain, sepsis, haemorrhage and post-surgical shock – had not been found. Of these, pain was the gravest handicap to the surgeon's task.

A few attempts were made at using 'mesmerism' to block out pain. The Scottish surgeon James Braid (1795–1861) showed that genuine sleep could be induced by staring fixedly at a bright object. Hypnosis was first used in surgical operations by John Elliotson (1791–1868), who published his results in 1843. Two years later, James Esdaile (1808–59) performed 261 painless operations (with only 5.5 per cent mortality) on Hindu prisoners in Bengal; but afterwards found that his fellow Scots were less susceptible to a state of trance.

Sleep-inducing drugs of various kinds have been used since the earliest days – including Homer's nepenthe, hemp in the East, and the mandrake concoction used by Hugh of Lucca in the thirteenth century. No single drug was consistently effective, and in Europe up to the middle of the last century the only relief for the agony of the operation was a large quantity of alcohol.

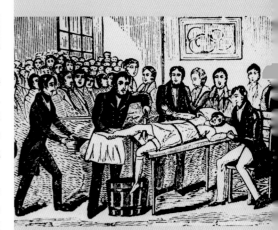

Above: an operation before anaesthesia – the patient is strapped to the operating table and held down by two strong men.

Right: the first successful public demonstration of anaesthesia, at Massachusetts General Hospital on 16 October 1846.

...144

Anaesthesia has the two functions of eliminating pain and inducing a state of muscular relaxation in the patient, thus making easier the task of the surgeon. Before its discovery surgeons attempted to overcome their difficulties by operating as speedily as possible. The problem of pain relief was solved not by the surgeons but by chemists. In 1772 Joseph Priestley discovered nitrous oxide: the analgesic and exhilarating effects of this gas were described in 1800 by Sir Humphry Davy, who suggested tentatively that it might be used with advantage in surgical operations.

The first person to prove that the pain of surgical operations could be abolished by the inhalation of gas was the English Henry Hill Hickman (1800–30). His discovery, which he published in 1824, was received without enthusiasm, and it was not until 1842 that modern surgical anaesthesia began, with the use of ether (the anaesthetic properties of which had been discovered by Faraday in 1818) by Crawford W Long (1815–78) of Jefferson, Georgia. His records state: 'James Venable, 1842, administration of ether and removal of tumour – 2 dollars'. Long, a modest country doctor, did not make known his results until 1849, by when he had used ether successfully a number of times and its effectiveness had been proved by the works of Morton and others.

William Thomas Green Morton (1819–68) first used ether at the Massachusetts General Hospital in 1846. Morton began his career in dentistry, then enrolled at the Harvard Medical School where the chemist Charles Jackson supplied him with ether and suggested he should try it to allay pain. On 30 September 1846, after experiments on dogs, Morton anaesthetized a patient before extracting a tooth and the news was published in the *Boston Daily Journal*. Then John Collins Warren, chief surgeon at the Massachusetts General Hospital, allowed Morton to try ether at the hospital. On 16 October 1846, Morton etherized a patient who then fell into a deep sleep, during which Warren excised a tumour of the neck. The patient work up shortly after the wound had been sutured and admitted that he had not felt any pain during the operation. The use of ether as an anaesthetic was publicized within a month and within another month it was being used in London.

Above: when Sir Humphry Davy first discovered the effects of inhaling nitrous oxide (laughing gas), it became a feature at parties for smart young people.

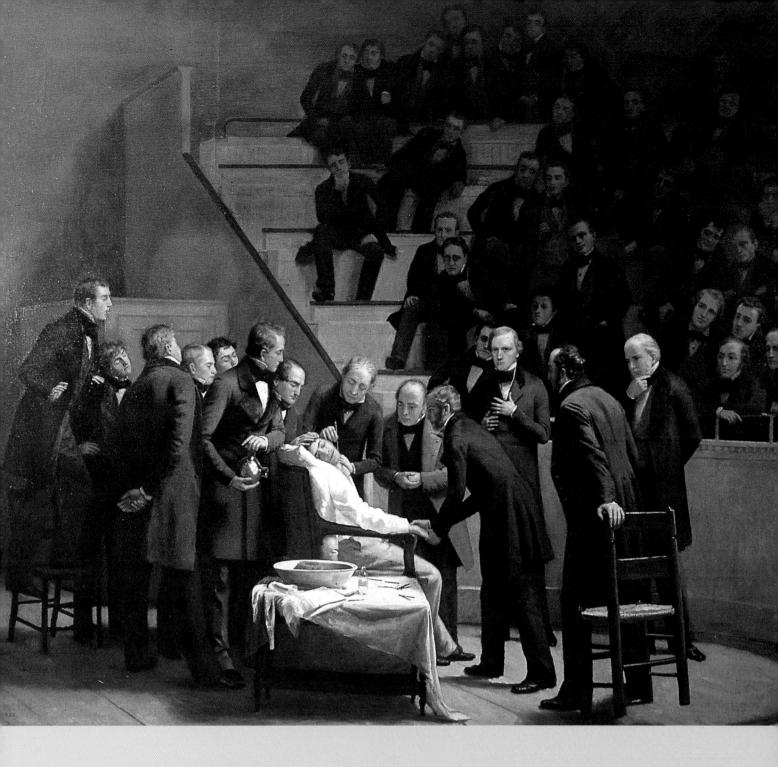

At the beginning of the nineteenth
century, surgery had limited horizons as
the solution of four difficult problems –
pain, sepsis, haemorrhage and post-
surgical shock – had not yet been found.
Of these, pain was the gravest handicap to
the surgeon's task.

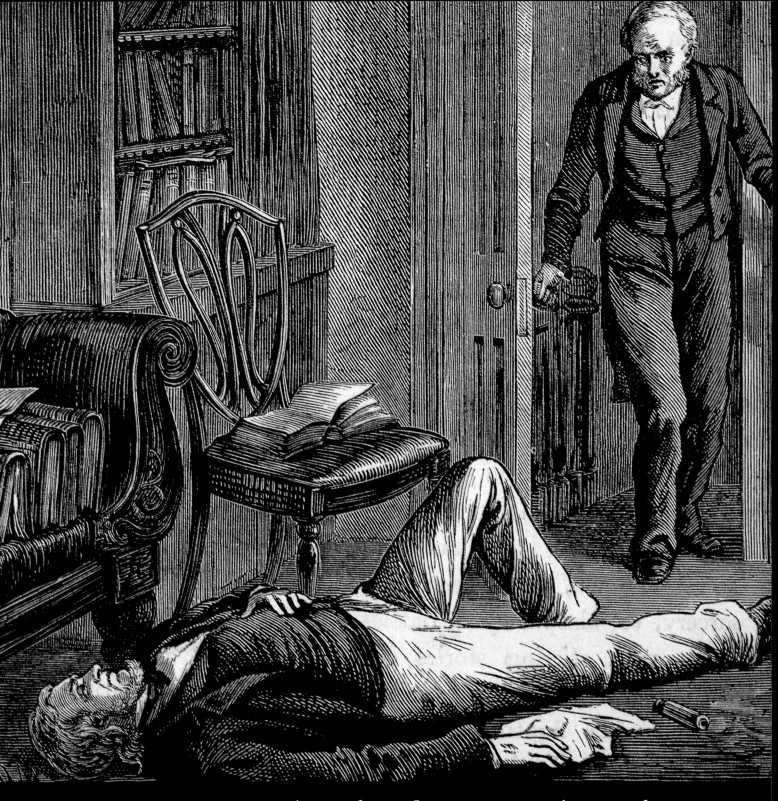

Above: Sir James Simpson experiments with chloroform in the early 1840s. He first used chloroform to relieve the pain of women during childbirth in 1847.

A number of names were given to the new discovery before the famous American clinician, Oliver Wendell Holmes, found an acceptable one – anaesthesia. The term was an ancient one derived from the Greek and meant insensitivity.

A number of names were given to the new discovery before the famous American clinician Oliver Wendell Holmes found an acceptable one: anaesthesia. The term was derived from the Greek and meant insensitivity, and was in fact an ancient one, used by Plato and Dioscorides.

When ether made its entry into Europe as a general anaesthetic at the end of 1846, the Scottish obstetrician Sir James Y Simpson (1811–70) was dissatisfied with its action because of its persistent and strong smell and the bronchial irritation it caused. After many experiments, he adopted a new anaesthetic, chloroform, which had been independently described by Eugène Soubeiran and Justus von Liebig in 1831. In November 1847, he informed the association of surgeons of Edinburgh about his discovery, thus incurring the wrath of the Scottish clergy. The Calvinists maintained that Genesis stated, 'with pangs shall you give birth to children'. Simpson replied by reminding his opponents that God made Adam fall into a deep sleep before taking the rib from him; in other words God anaesthetized him. When some doctors of Philadelphia wrote to him protesting that the pain of childbirth, as a spontaneous, natural and therefore necessary manifestation, should not be eliminated, Simpson advised them not to take the train next time they went to New York, if they wished to be spontaneous and natural, but make the journey on foot. Simpson's victory was complete when Queen Victoria requested administration of an anaesthetic for the delivery of Prince Leopold, her seventh child. With royal assent, anaesthesia became at once fashionable and acceptable.

Anaesthesia was quickly adopted in every hospital. Technical developments and the introduction of new anaesthetics helped to overcome some of the initial difficulties. Ether irritated the respiratory tract. Chloroform could damage the liver and cardiac muscle and cause circulatory failure. A mixture of oxygen and nitrous oxide was less toxic, but this did not produce deep narcosis or sufficient muscle relaxation. The action of ethyl chloride (introduced in 1848) was too short-lived. Surgeons needed an anaesthetic that was not only non-toxic but also non-inflammable, for new electric surgical instruments were introduced in operating theatres, and these made sparks which could lead to an explosion in atmospheres impregnated with the vapour of the anaesthetic. Of the new anaesthetics, cyclopropane, introduced in 1929, had the disadvantage of being readily inflammable; trichloroethylene was first used in 1934, and was found to have the twofold advantage of reducing awareness of pain without eliminating consciousness, and was thus suitable for use in childbirth.

Intravenous anaesthesia was first achieved by Pierre Cyprien Oré (1828–89) of Bordeaux in 1874, using chloral, but came into general use after 1902 when Emil Fischer performed the synthesis of Veronal. After Veronal, many other barbiturates were introduced, and of these thiopentone is generally used today for the induction of anaesthesia. These substances have a very effective sedative action but do not produce insensibility to pain, so they have been used in association with other anaesthetics.

147...

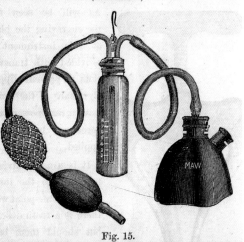

(Junker's.)

Fig. 15.

Left: the Junker inhaler, invented in 1867 and still in use in the early twentieth century.

After 1945 two other drugs came into use in anaesthesia: curare and succinyl-choline, both of which produce muscular relaxation. South American Indians poison their arrows with curare: the prey, wounded but not killed, is unable to escape because its muscles are paralysed by the poison. The curare used in anaesthesia is tubocurarine, one of the active principles extracted from the bark of *Strychnos toxifera*.

Another type of anaesthesia, in many instances much more advantageous for the patient, had long been sought by surgeons: local anaesthesia. This was achieved in 1884 by the Austrian Karl Koller (1857–1944) using cocaine. Today cocaine is used only in eye and throat operations but the drug is only really effective when applied to surfaces, and, for other procedures, more effective and less toxic substances, such as procaine and lignocaine, are preferred. Local analgesia has the advantage of sparing the patient any unpleasant side-effects. Again, it enables operations to be carried out that would not be possible under general anaesthesia. Local anaesthesia is often combined with the use of a hypnotic (a drug to induce sleep).

In 1898 August Karl Gustav Bier (1861–1949) of Greifswald injected cocaine into the vertebral canal and obtained analgesia of the lower extremities; then he used the method in surgical operations, and since then spinal anaesthesia has become widely used. Another method of administering anaesthetics was first achieved in 1847 by the Russian surgeon Nikolai Ivanovich Pirogov (1810–81), who introduced ether into the rectum; this substance proved too irritant and other substances are now in general use.

Anaesthesia has been a speciality of medicine for over a century. The task of the anaesthetist is a complex one, for he must not only administer and regulate the anaesthetic but also control respiration at every moment of the operation, especially when the patient has been given drugs that, like curare, cause relaxation of all the muscles (including those of respiration). In addition, the anaesthetist must at all times be prepared to intervene with suitable drugs to correct any excessive fall or rise in blood pressure, and indeed with these drugs to alter the blood pressure if bleeding becomes excessive or the patient shocked.

...148

Below: an anaesthetist administers an epidural anaesthetic to a pregnant woman before the delivery of her baby. A local anaesthetic is injected into the epidural space around the membranes surrounding the spinal cord, to relieve pain in the lower part of the body.

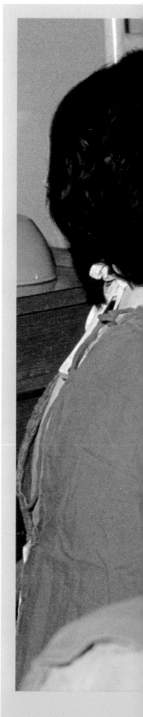

Since the Second World War, new techniques for the administration of anaesthesia have been developed, such as spinal injection to produce anaesthesia of the lower part of the body, for use in child birth. Later it was replaced by epidural anaesthesia, which requires the services of a skilled anaesthetist.

The modern anaesthetist is equipped with a range of skills including techniques to induce safe anaesthesia, using sophisticated machines such as heart-lung bypass machines, and the use of intensive care suites to ensure recovery from major operations, accidents and illnesses. Recent advances in epidural anaesthesia and spinal blocks have helped patients who may previously have been considered unfit for a general anaesthetic. The development of these skills seems to have led naturally to anaesthetists taking a major role as pain management experts. Since the first pain clinic opened in Seattle in 1946, pain clinics have come into existence in most developed countries. Patients receive drug therapy, acupuncture, instruction in relaxation techniques and counselling to improve the quality of their lives. Many pain clinics now include a specially trained anaesthetist who can give advice on a variety of pain control techniques and can perform nerve blocks and other treatments which improve the lives of many long-term pain sufferers.

149...

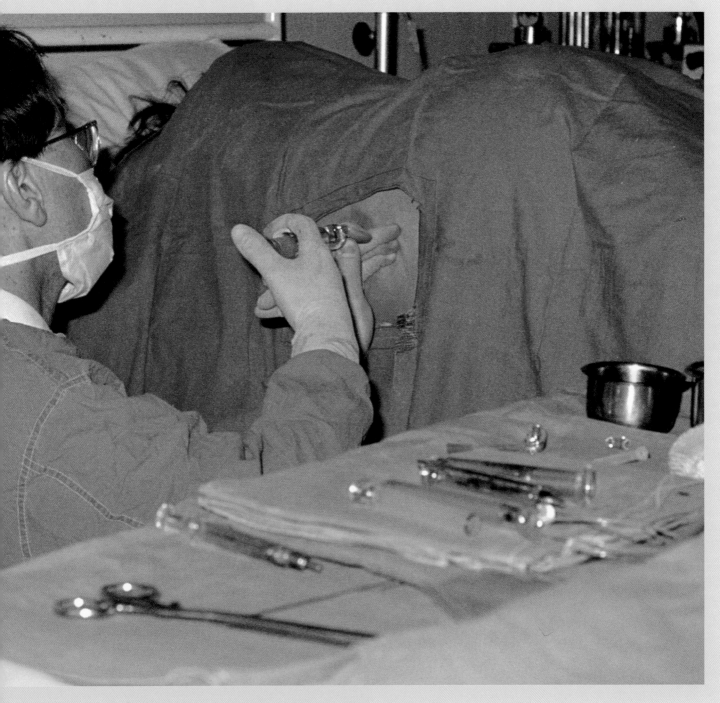

MILITARY MEDICINE AND NURSING

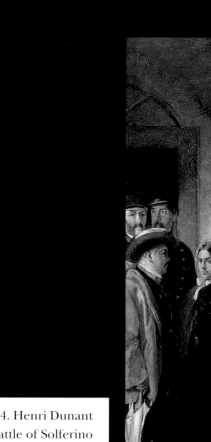

In centuries of warfare armies have been defeated as often by epidemic diseases as by battle wounds, for the destructive effect of war on hygiene and order has always favoured the spread of infections. Military medicine, aiming to treat the sick as well as the wounded soldier, developed slowly. Only at the end of the eighteenth century were the first permanent medical corps formed and army hospitals and field stations established. It is impossible to estimate what proportion of the 6,000,000 French and allied soldiers lost in the Napoleonic Wars died in battle or from their wounds and what proportion from other causes; but this loss was a physical disaster of the first magnitude for France and brought home the need for really efficient medical care in wartime. The Crimean War emphasized this for the Allies, for wretched hospital standards – later raised by Florence Nightingale's work – resulted in enormous and unnecessary losses. The same happened in the American Civil War, in which over twice as many soldiers died from disease as from battle wounds.

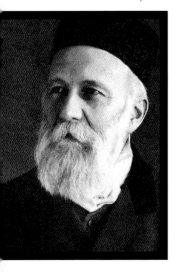

The event which was to alter this picture occurred in 1864. Henri Dunant (1828–1910), a Swiss philanthropist, who was present at the battle of Solferino was so outraged and moved by the sufferings of the wounded that he wrote his *Souvenir de Solferino*, which was published in 1862. This aroused such popular support that an International Conference of Red Cross Societies, each a national organization formed to aid the wounded of its country, was held in Geneva in 1863. Following this, on 22 August 1864, fourteen nations signed agreement to the Geneva Convention: according to the Convention, all sick and wounded, as well as the army medical and nursing staffs, were to be treated as neutrals on the battlefield. The Red Cross movement was widely supported from its inception, and today every country has its Red Cross Society to give relief in times of flood, famine and earthquake as well as war.

Not only the Red Cross, but advances in preventive medicine have improved the lot of the soldier. Vaccination and immunization have played an

Above: Henri Dunant,
the founder of the
Red Cross.

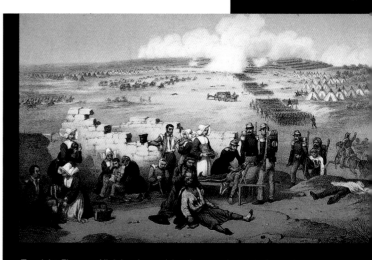

Top right: Florence Nightingale receiving the wounded at the barrack hospital in Scutari, 1856.

Above: a field hospital at the battle of Inkerman, 1854, one of the battles during the siege of Sebastopol during the Crimean War.

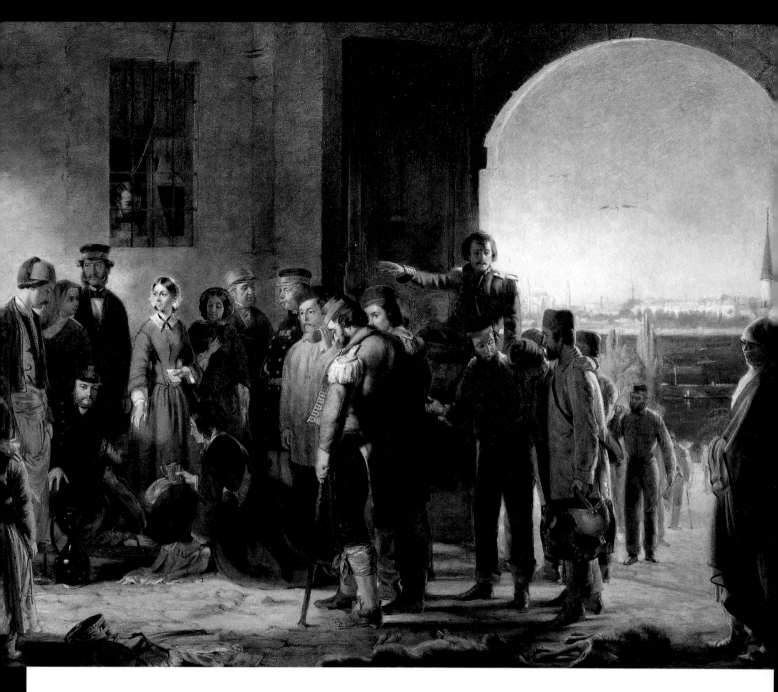

important part, as was shown by the incidence of smallpox in the Franco-Prussian War in 1870–71. The historian Fielding Garrison notes that there were only 483 cases among the vaccinated German troops, while the largely unvacci-nated French had 4,178, with 2,000 fatalities. In addition, proper asepsis and good nursing gave the Germans advantage over their opponents.

Perhaps the most famous figure in the history of nursing was Florence Nightingale. Born in Florence, Italy, in 1823, into an upper-class English family, she devoted her whole life to nursing, and her reforms were fundamental in making it the admirable institution it is today. A woman of immensely strong will, in March 1854, at the outbreak of the Crimean War, she persuaded Sidney Herbert, the Secretary of War, to let her go with some of her nurses to take charge of the barrack hospital at Scutari, where her tireless care for the wounded and sick at all hours won her the affectionate title of the 'lady with the lamp'. Florence Nightingale's work was so successful that on her return to England £50,000 was raised to establish a school for nurses at St Thomas's Hospital, London, which was opened on 15 June 1860.

ANTISEPSIS AND ASEPSIS

In the first half of the nineteenth century, infection of wounds very frequently complicated surgical operations, and led to disaster in cases which might otherwise have been successfully treated. After operations, healing of wounds by first intent, that is with scar formation unaccompanied by an inflammatory response, was very unusual. So great was the toll of infection that mortality amounted to 45 per cent in cases of amputation. After the operation, the patient faced not only secondary haemorrhage but also tetanus, erysipelas and septicaemia. Innumerable women died of puerperal sepsis a few days after giving birth. The cause of the high death rate in the surgical wards of the hospitals was still unknown at the middle of the last century. It was often thought that it was something in the air, a poisonous vapour.

If the cause of pus formation and inflammation was still obscure, the mechanism of these processes began to be understood at this time. Simpson of St Andrews was the first to suggest (in 1722) that pus came from capillaries, and this was confirmed by observations of Augustus Waller and Thomas Addison (1849) and by the work of Julius Cohnheim.

The theory of poisonous vapour was disproved by the Hungarian obstetrician Ignaz Philipp Semmelweiss (1818–65). After studying at the university of Vienna, in 1846 he joined the staff on maternity ward No 1 at the Vienna Krankenhaus as assistant to a well-known obstetrician. He was at once disturbed by the many deaths among the newly delivered women: in his first month in his department, thirty-six died out of a total of 208. In search of clues to this disastrous mortality, Semmelweiss observed that in one year, 1846, the number of deaths in maternity ward No 1 was of the order of 451, whereas in ward No 2 there were only ninety deaths from puerperal fever. It seemed unlikely that the hypothetical 'invisible vapour' in ward No 1 was more of a killer than in ward No 2. His attention was drawn to the post-mortem room; it was then the custom for obstetricians to carry out autopsies early in the day and then go on with their ward work. The post-mortem room and the number of deaths seemed to be connected; for the second ward, where deaths were far less frequent, was staffed by midwives who never attended autopsies.

In 1847 returned Semmelweiss from a brief holiday to find that his colleague Kolletschka had died from septicaemia after cutting himself with a scalpel during an autopsy. He attended the post mortem and noted that the lesions were similar to those he had observed on so many occasions in women with puerperal fever. It was the scalpel that had transferred the 'invisible poison' from the corpse to Kolletschka.

Convinced that the infection was transmitted in this way, Semmelweiss issued stringent orders: before visiting a patient, everyone was to wash his hands carefully and the wards were to be cleaned with calcium chloride. After this the mortality rate from puerperal fever in ward No 1 dropped dramatically from 12 per cent to almost zero within two years. Semmelweiss then communicated these findings to the medical society in Vienna; and was instantly attacked by almost all his colleagues. Despite the support of three senior non-obstetrical professors, he was dismissed from his post and returned embittered to Budapest. In the maternity ward No 1 doctors and students stopped washing and disinfecting their hands after autopsies and the death rate among the

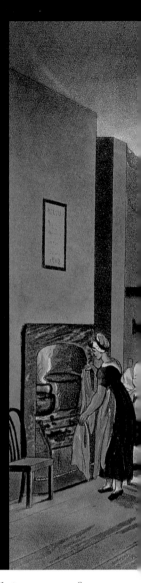

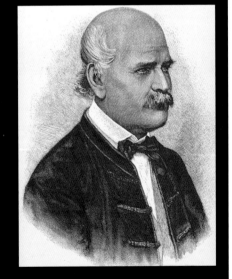

Above: Ignaz Semmelweiss, the Hungarian obstetrician whose sterling work was met with derision from his superiors.

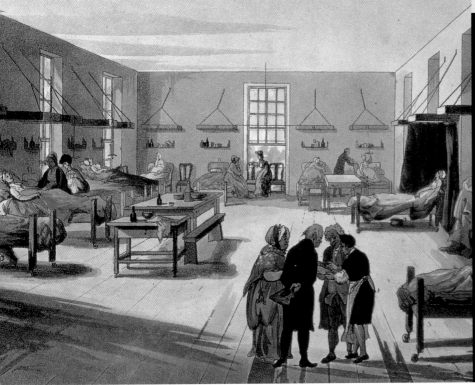

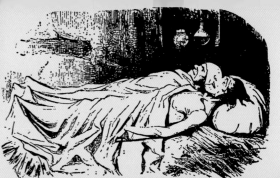

153...

Surgical pain had been overcome by the
discovery of anaesthetics, but the problem
of infection continued to complicate the
tasks of surgeons and physicians. It was the
pioneering work of a Hungarian
obstetrician, Ignaz Semmelweiss, which
showed that the fever that killed many
women after childbirth was carried on dirty
hands and instruments and could be
banished by cleanliness and antiseptics.

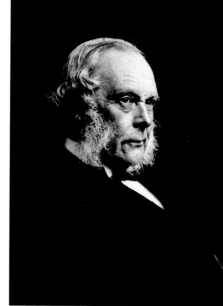

Right: Joseph Lister, whose practical steps to cut down on the spread of infection in hospitals were rewarded with the highest honours.

...154

newly delivered women returned to its old level. In Hungary, Semmelweiss continued to practise antisepsis and succeeded in removing puerperal sepsis from the maternity ward of the old hospital of St Roch in Budapest.

Ultimately Semmelweiss published his work *Die Aetiologie, der Begriff und die Prophylaxis des Kindbettfiebers* (1861), which stands as one of the epoch-making books of medical literature. However, it is extremely difficult to read, with a mass of barely comprehensible statistics, and was received with unrelieved hostility by the medical profession. It was twenty years before Semmelweiss's ideas were to be accepted and later still, in 1894, before a monument was erected to him in Budapest.

Joseph Lister, one of the greatest names in the history of surgery, introduced disinfection to the hospital at Glasgow at the time when Semmelweiss's work was rejected. Lister (1827–1912) had been a student of the famous surgeon James Syme in Edinburgh and was already familiar with Pasteur's work on micro-organisms when he started to work on antisepsis. Determined to reduce post-operative infections and hospital gangrene, he adopted disinfection – one of the three ways Pasteur had shown to combat the growth of micro-organisms. He insisted on meticulous cleanliness of his wards and instruments and the patients' dressings, and used a variety of antiseptics before selecting carbolic acid (phenol), which he tried out on cases of compound fracture. He had observed that simple fractures healed without complications, whereas those accompanied by laceration of the skin were subject to suppuration and gangrene. The skin was thus an effective barrier against infection, the agents of which were presumably pathogenic bacteria, although this was not yet proven. Thus another barrier, a chemical one, was needed as a replacement when the skin was broken. Lister's system was simple: he treated the wound with carbolic acid then placed a piece of linen, also soaked in dilute phenol, on top of the wound, and secured it with plaster; he then covered the dressing with metal foil to reduce evaporation of the antiseptic. Before starting an operation, Lister had carbolic acid sprayed in the operating theatre and so disinfected not only the instruments but the operative field of the patient's skin as well. He first used this method on 12 August 1865, and he published his results in a series of articles in the *Lancet* in 1867. Lister's results were so strikingly good that the new method caught on at once and spread all over the world.

At this time, a great many surgeons were famous for their technical ability and the speed with which they operated. In contrast, Lister became famous

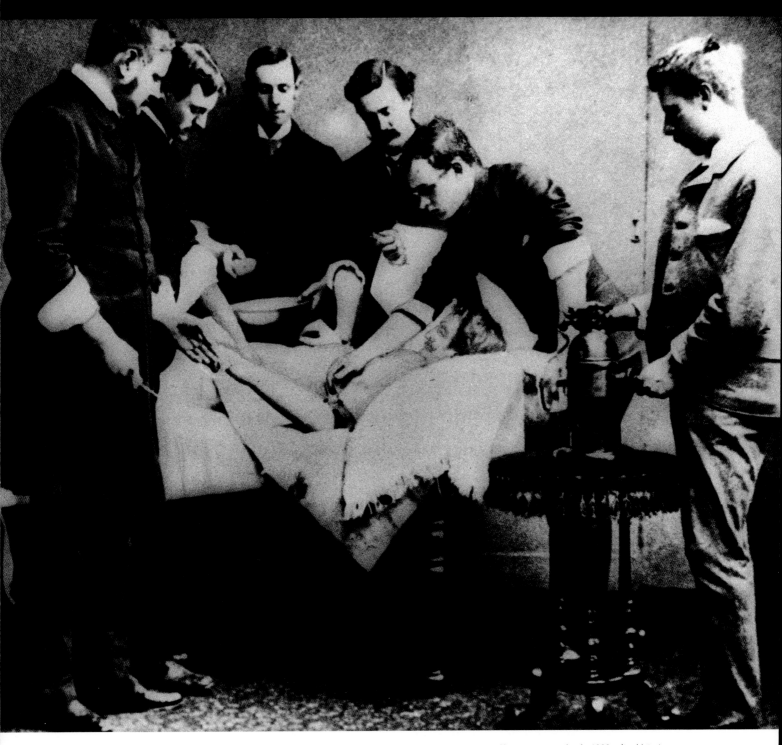

because most of his patients survived the operations and recovered within a short period of time without complications. Antisepsis and anaesthesia between them changed the whole nature of surgery. His work was rewarded with the highest honours and in 1897 he was raised to the peerage, thus becoming the first doctor to sit in the House of Lords.

The era of antisepsis was followed by the era of asepsis. At a certain point surgeons felt hampered by antiseptics; instead of destroying micro-organisms and at the same time damaging the patient's tissues, they aimed to exclude bacteria totally from the operating theatre. Asepsis made use of another of Pasteur's combative measures – heat. In 1886 the German Ernst von Bergmann (1836–1907) introduced steam sterilization of dressings, and four years later the American W S Halsted (1852–1922) initiated the use of sterile rubber gloves during operations.

Above: an operation in 1883, after Lister's antiseptic methods had become widely established. The hand-operated phenol spray is on the table to the right of the picture.

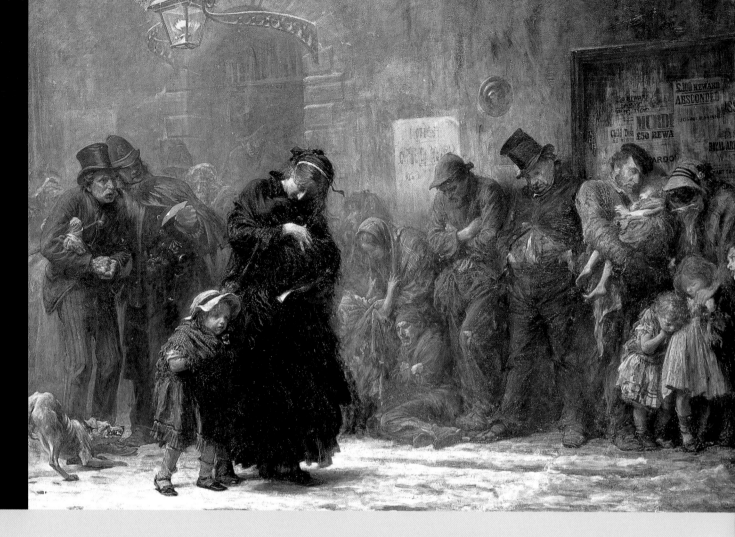

PUBLIC HEALTH

Above: Awaiting Admission to the Casual Ward by Sir Luke Fildes. Fildes made his name when this picture, vividly expressing the sufferings of the poor, was exhibited at the Academy in 1874, when he was only thirty.

Many of the landmarks of public health through the ages have already been described in this book, from the sewer system of ancient Rome to the reform of hospitals by Florence Nightingale and Lord Lister.

One of the greatest problems facing large cities was the disposal of solid excreta. As late as the eighteenth century faeces and urine were thrown into the streets, and in London the excreta were collected and dumped in refuse piles. Unfortunately refuse was flushed into cesspools whose contents soaked into the earth, thus polluting wells, or were drained into rivers; in London, the Thames and Serpentine became no better than open sewers. Even in better-class houses, water closets did not became general until about 1830.

Particularly in the rapidly growing manufacturing towns of the north, the Industrial Revolution produced hundreds of thousands of jerry-built hovels in which disease was favoured by lack of ventilation and light, in addition to over-crowding. The importance of fresh air under such conditions was realized early. Stephen Hales (1677–1761) devised in 1743 a ventilator by means of which fresh air could get into prisons, the holds of ships, mines and other confined spaces. This invention was at once widely used, producing improvement in health and living conditions.

The repeal of the evil window tax in 1803 helped a little with light and ventilation, but in smoky industrial towns there was little enough light, and this, combined with the poverty of the urban diet in comparison with that of the country people, resulted in rickets, 'the English disease'. People were still unaware that there were such things as deficiency diseases, although scurvy was successfully treated with citrus fruit in 1747 by James Lind (1716–94).

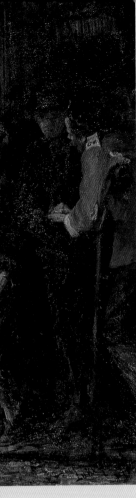

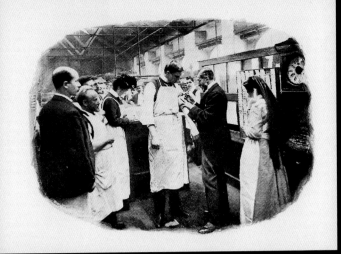

This new era really began with the work of Sir Edwin Chadwick, through whose efforts the Public Health Act of 1848 was passed. Determined to improve the lot of the working classes in the large towns, he prepared a report on their sanitary conditions and showed why mortality was greatest in the slums; his findings revealed such a distressing picture that they were received by Parliament 'with astonishment, dismay, horror and even incredulity'. The Act of 1848 put into practice for the first time the principle that a state was responsible for the health of its people. One of Chadwick's innovations was the use of glazed earthenware pipes for sewage, which reduced the possibility of contamination of drinking water. At the same time it was decided that shallow wells should be abolished and mains water supply introduced. This was partly thanks to the detective work of the anaesthetist John Snow, who collected data on a number of outbreaks of cholera and showed the disease to be water-borne.

The cholera pandemics began in the early 1830s and produced great apprehension as well as a good deal of thorough epidemiological investigation. The official report on the first outbreak in Paris in 1832 began 'When a deadly scourge, such a famine, pestilence, or an epidemic strikes a great city, the first feeling that it arouses is terror. Everyone has but one thought, one object: to escape the evil. Those whose position or wealth allows it flee in all haste; those – and they are in the majority – for whom flight is impossible, forced to remain, give way to fatal despondency.' One particularly severe outbreak occurred in Soho, London, in 1854, with 14,000 cases and 618 deaths; Snow suggested that an invisible living agent was responsible and traced the infection to a well in Broad (now Broadwick) Street, an appallingly overcrowded area, which was contaminated from a leaking cesspool.

Thus, during the second half of the nineteenth century the efforts of the state were directed at improvement of the physical environment rather than at implementing the recent advances in medicine at the individual level. That preventive medicine alone was not enough in reducing disease in the poor was revealed forcibly at the end of the century, when the alarming discovery was made that half of the army recruits for service in South Africa were physically unfit. It became increasingly recognized that poverty and everything that went with it predisposed strongly to disease. The state awoke to this dangerous situation in time for the Great War, introducing school meals, the School Medical Service (1907) and the National Insurance Act of 1911. This provided free medical services for many of the working population, and was based on a system that had been established successfully in Germany. It marked the beginnings of state medicine and presaged the five acts of 1944–48 which provided a comprehensive system of social security for everyone in Great Britain.

The new era began with the work of Sir Edwin Chadwick, through whose efforts the Public Health Act of 1848 was passed.

VICTORY OVER INFECTION

In the second half of the nineteenth century, revolutionary developments in microbiology had a profound effect both on knowledge of the causes and effects of disease and the approach of doctors to illness. In Germany especially, the leading clinicians began to attach the greatest importance to laboratory investigation, sometimes to the detriment of clinical observation. Since Germany then led the world, clinical medicine in some other countries began to take second place to laboratory research.

The foundations of scientific medicine in Germany were laid by Johannes Müller (1801–58), an able investigator in many fields. Among his achievements were studies of colour vision, sensation and speech, while through his influence on such pupils as Schwann, Henle, Kölliker, Virchow, Du-Bois Reymond, Helmholtz and Brücke, as Garrison remarked, 'we may trace the main currents of modern German medicine'. Jakob Henle (1809–85) discoverer of the renal tubules that bear his name, was among the first to uphold that micro-organisms caused infectious disease. In his treatise *On Miasms and Contagions*, he wrote 'the substance of contagion is not only organic but living, and endowed with a life of its own, which has a parasitic relation to the sick body'.

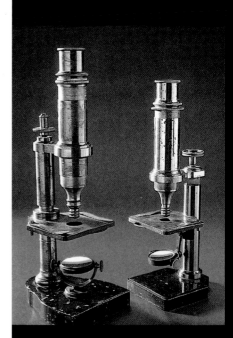

Above: microscopes used by Louis Pasteur, and designed by Joseph Jackson Lister, father of Joseph Lister and an amateur microscopist.

...158 **The greatest nineteenth-century pathologist was Rudolph Virchow, who stated that diseases were manifested in the cells and not in invisible and intangible humours.**

Rudolf Ludwig Karl Virchow (1821–1902) dominated medicine for more than half of the nineteenth century and is undoubtedly one of the greatest pathologists. He studied medicine at the university of Berlin and in 1846 began to teach pathological anatomy, writing that 'pathological anatomy and clinical medicine, the justification and independence of which we fully recognize, have particular value for us as the source of new problems, the answers to which belong to physio-pathology'. In 1849 he went to Silesia to study an epidemic of exanthematous typhus and published an indignant account of the miserable conditions in which the workers lived; this account, which characterized his freedom of political utterance, displeased the authorities and he was forced to resign. He spent seven years at Würzburg, during which he laid the foundations of his great work, and then returned to Berlin where he became professor and director of the Institute of Pathological Anatomy of the Charité Hospital, a post he held until 1902, the year of his death.

In 1858 he published his great work, *Die cellularpathologie*, in which he asserted that the seat of disease should always be sought in the cell, while the macroscopic and microscopic changes in the organism in disease were the reaction of cells to the cause of disease. This doctrine opened the way for the microscopic study of tissues and at the same time replaced for ever the old idea that diseases were caused by invisible and intangible humours. He later wrote: 'The essence of disease, according to my idea, is a modified part of the organism or rather a modified cell or aggregation of cells (whether of tissue or of organs). . . . In fact every diseased part of the body holds a parasitic relation to the rest of the healthy body to which it belongs, and it lives at the expense of the organism.'

At the time when he founded his doctrine Virchow did not know the nature of the extraneous forces which he held responsible for many diseased states. This was explained by Louis Pasteur, who showed that micro-organisms caused disease and themselves came from micro-organisms, thereby demolishing for ever the theory of spontaneous generation.

'In the field of observation, events favour only those who are prepared': stated Pasteur during his inaugural lecture at the university of Lille.

The son of a tanner, Louis Pasteur was born on 27 December 1822 at Dôle in the Jura. From the college at Besançon he went to Paris to study chemistry and then to teaching posts at Dijon, Strasbourg and Lille. In his inaugural lecture at the university of Lille he made his famous remark: 'In the field of observation, events favour only those who are prepared', which so often applied to his discoveries. In 1857 he became director of scientific studies at the Paris Ecole Normale and his most important work began.

He was asked by a wine company to study fermentation, then thought to be caused by the breakdown of dead yeast. Pasteur showed, on the contrary, that it was produced by living micro-organisms. He ascertained that yeasts in sugar solution took up oxygen from the air and multiplied rapidly, producing little alcohol. Introduced into the same solution but not exposed to air, the organisms utilized the oxygen in the sugar, liberating a large quantity of alcohol. Pasteur also found that vinegar was the product of the decomposition of wine, caused by living organisms; and that milk, similarly, became lactic acid. This was called fermentation when the product was useful and putrefaction when it was harmful. His discovery of the lactic acid bacilli was soon followed by that of the bacteria responsible for butyric acid fermentation. These could not only live without oxygen but actually flourished in an atmosphere of carbon dioxide, and were thus 'anaerobic' as distinct from 'aerobic' organisms.

159...

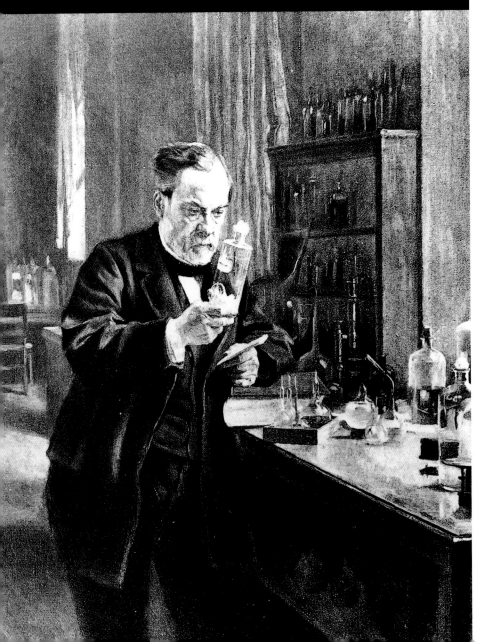

Left: Louis Pasteur at work in his laboratory, by Albert Edelfelt

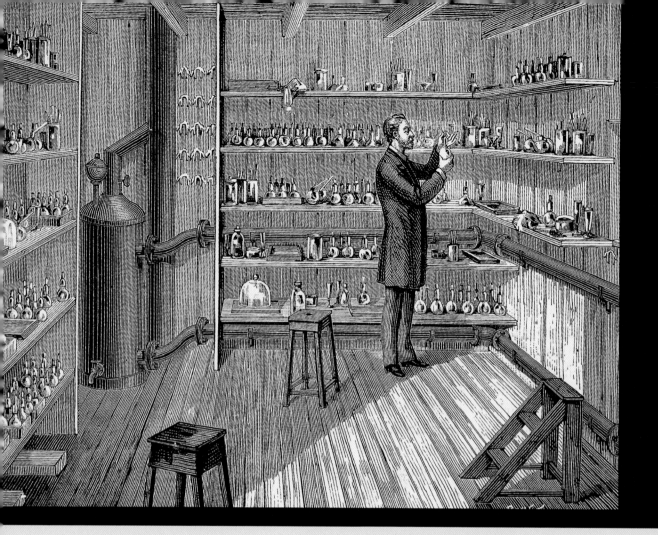

Above: a hot room for the cultivation of microbes at the Institut Pasteur in Paris, circa 1890.

In 1864 Pasteur was invited by the same wine producers to investigate the reasons for the souring of wine and to suggest a remedy. He discovered that bacteria-free fluids remained free of bacteria if properly protected, and one of the means of protection was heat; he showed that heating the wine for a short while to 60°C (108°F) killed the organism (*Mycetum aceti*) that was responsible for the formation of vinegar without affecting the quality of the wine. This system was also applied to other products and came to be known as pasteurization. In 1865, Pasteur saved the French silk industry from ruin, by throwing light on pébrine, a disease that was destroying silk worms. He next studied cholera in chickens, a disease that was raging in epidemic form in several parts of France. He succeeded in isolating the pathogenic organism and discovered that old cultures lost their virulence and that when injected into poultry made them immune from virulent germs. This 'attenuation' of the organism made immunization possible against other diseases.

He studied anthrax, an infectious disease of cattle and horses which was transmitted to man through infected meat or hides. He made the causative bacilli less virulent by heating them to a temperature of 42°C (75.6°F) and then inoculating sheep with them; when the sheep were subsequently injected with virulent bacilli, they did not develop anthrax. In the spring of 1881, Pasteur repeated his experiments in public at Melun with forty-eight sheep, injecting virulent anthrax bacilli into twenty-four sheep previously immunized with an injection of a culture of attenuated bacilli and twenty-four sheep not thus immunized. After forty-eight hours, twenty-two of the second group were dead, whereas all the vaccinated animals were perfectly healthy.

Although he had a stroke which left his left side partly paralysed, Pasteur continued his memorable work, and as his final achievement discovered a means of treating rabies. Two rabid dogs were brought to his laboratory, and he discovered that the rabies virus was present not only in the saliva but in the nervous systems of the sick animals, and could be attenuated by drying the spinal cord. He injected healthy animals with a suspension of nervous tissue from infected dogs and demonstrated to a government commission that they were immune from rabies.

In the summer of 1885, a woman came to him from Alsace with her nine-year-old son, Joseph Meister, who had been bitten by a rabid dog two days earlier. The disease would have developed in the child from three to six weeks after the dog bite, the symptoms including fever, malaise, nausea and a sore throat, then spasms of the muscles of mouth and throat, at first on drinking but later at the mere sight of fluid (hence the name hydrophobia), followed by severe spasms and convulsions, maniacal behaviour, and finally paralysis, coma and death. On 16 July, ten days after the boy had come to him, Pasteur began inoculation with a suspension of dried spinal cord of rabbits which had been infected with rabies. On 26 October, he was able to inform the Académie des Sciences that Joseph Meister was safe.

Pasteur's last achievement was received with great enthusiasm, and the Institut Pasteur was set up in Paris to enable him to continue his work in discovering new pathogenic agents and preparing new cultures for immunization against disease. There he worked tirelessly to the end of his life, gathering around him a school of famous pupils. Universally honoured and recognized throughout the world as a great scientist and benefactor of mankind, he died at the age of seventy-three in September 1895.

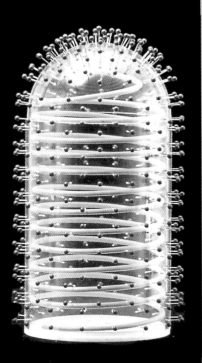

Above: a structural model of a rhabdovirus particle, the virus that causes rabies.

Below: Pasteur supervising a session of anti-rabies vaccinations.

161...

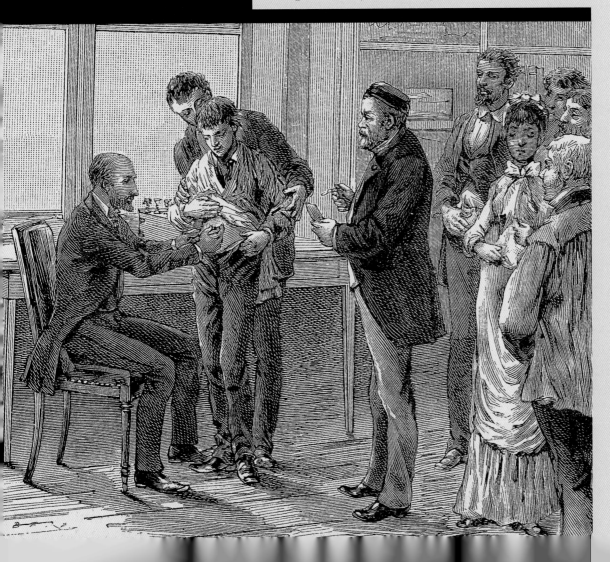

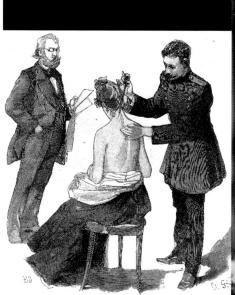

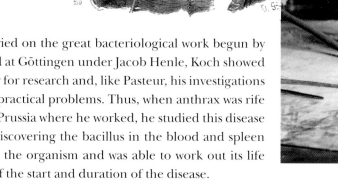

Right: Robert Koch, on the left, supervising an injection during the course of treatment for tuberculosis, 1891.

Robert Koch (1843–1910) carried on the great bacteriological work begun by Pasteur. A German who studied at Göttingen under Jacob Henle, Koch showed an extraordinary technical flair for research and, like Pasteur, his investigations were stimulated by immediate practical problems. Thus, when anthrax was rife among the stock in the part of Prussia where he worked, he studied this disease intensively and succeeded in discovering the bacillus in the blood and spleen of a dead animal. He cultured the organism and was able to work out its life cycle and clarify the question of the start and duration of the disease.

Koch carried Pasteur's work further with his own great discovery of the tubercle bacillus, the organism causing tuberculosis. This bacillus has a waxy coat which makes it difficult to stain by methods which suffice for other bacteria, and it is also a difficult one to culture. Koch's work extended the field of bacteriology by introducing new methods of staining, to make more organisms visible under the microscope, and also new ways of culturing bacteria. With these new methods, Koch was able to succeed with *Mycobacterium tuberculosis*, where others had failed, and his work won him the highest honours, including the Nobel prize in 1905.

In 1868 the French pathologist Jean Antoine Villemin had demonstrated the main features of the morbid anatomy of tuberculosis and had shown that the disease was transmissible in animals by means of tuberculous material. In 1882 Koch cultivated the tubercle bacillus, and presented his results to the Berlin Physiological Society in a paper which also included 'Koch's postulates': 1, that the organism must always be found in a given disease; 2, that the organism must not be found in other diseases or in health; 3, that the organism must be cultivated artificially and reproduce the given disease after the inoculation of a pure culture into a susceptible animal; 4, that the organism must be recoverable from the animal so inoculated. This set of rules must be followed if it is to be proved that a specified organism is responsible for a specific disease.

Paul Ehrlich (1854–1915) was an outstanding scientific genius who produced the scientific basis for immunology and founded chemotherapy. The son of a Jewish merchant from Strehlen in Silesia, he studied at Strasbourg and Freiburg before qualifying at Leipzig in 1878. Even as a student Ehrlich experi-

Paul Ehrlich was the founder of immunology. He prepared substances, such as salvarsan, whose toxic effects on bacteria were far greater than on the human body.

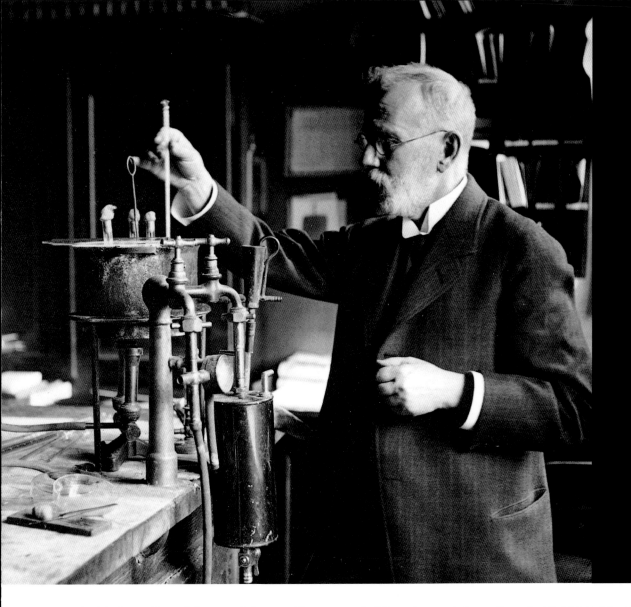

Above: Paul Ehrlich in his laboratory. In 1908 he shared the Nobel prize with Elie Metchnikoff for work on immunology.

mented with dyestuffs and tissue staining, and he wrote a brilliant doctoral thesis on the staining of histological specimens for examination under the microscope. He showed that some of the white blood cells were selectively stained by basic dyes, that the urine of typhoid patients reacted with diazo dyes, and that tubercle bacilli retained the colour of carbol fuchsin after treatment with acid. His work led him to believe that certain tissues had an elective affinity for certain chemical substances and certain staining materials.

Ehrlich argued that if various tissues have specific components to which dyes are attached, it ought to be possible to make dyes perform tasks in various parts of the body. Thus to ascertain that an anaesthetic reached nervous tissue, all that would be necessary would be to colour it with methylene blue. He also formulated the hypothesis that dyes, as well as having an affinity for specific tissues, could select pathogenic micro-organisms. By studying trypanosomes, the parasites transmitted by the tsetse fly and causing sleeping sickness, he found the dye trypan red, which has some effect against these organisms.

In 1910, Ehrlich discovered salvarsan. This compound was known as 606 because it was the six hundred and sixth arsenical product to be synthesized in his chemotherapeutic institute, founded three years earlier. Although a great advance, neither salvarsan nor neosalvarsan, '914', was successful in conquering syphilis; that victory was won by penicillin.

Ehrlich's work on immunity laid the foundations for the science of immunology. The actions of antibodies on harmful organisms were worked out by others. Thus Richard Pfeiffer (1858–1945) showed that in a guinea pig that had been immunized against cholera, the vibrios that caused the disease, when injected into the peritoneal cavity, were dissolved (bacteriolysis). The substances responsible for this process, bacteriolysins, were antibodies to the antigens of the cholera. In the reaction between antigen and antibody, 'complement', a substance also present in normal serum, was used up. This applied not only to bacteriolysis but also to such phenomena as agglutination and haemolysis, seen after transfusion of incompatible blood. Complement fixation, as this was called, was studied by Jean Baptiste Vincent Bordet (1870–1961), who with Octave Gengou (1875–1959) worked out the complement fixation test which formed the basis not only for the Wasserman reaction but also for such diseases as gonorrhoea and glanders.

It followed that there were two possible means of protecting an individual against the effect of pathogenic organisms: active immunization, whereby a living organism of reduced virulence was introduced, and the individual manufactured his own antibodies in response to it, and passive immunization, whereby antibodies were given, in serum from an animal that had been infected. Jenner's work, of course, was the pioneer achievement in the former of these, while Pasteur had fought anthrax and rabies in the same way and Koch's tuberculin produced an active immune response. In the field of passive immunity, Behring and Kitasato's work was followed by treatments against plague and also the development of diagnostic tests for such conditions as diphtheria (the Schick test, 1913).

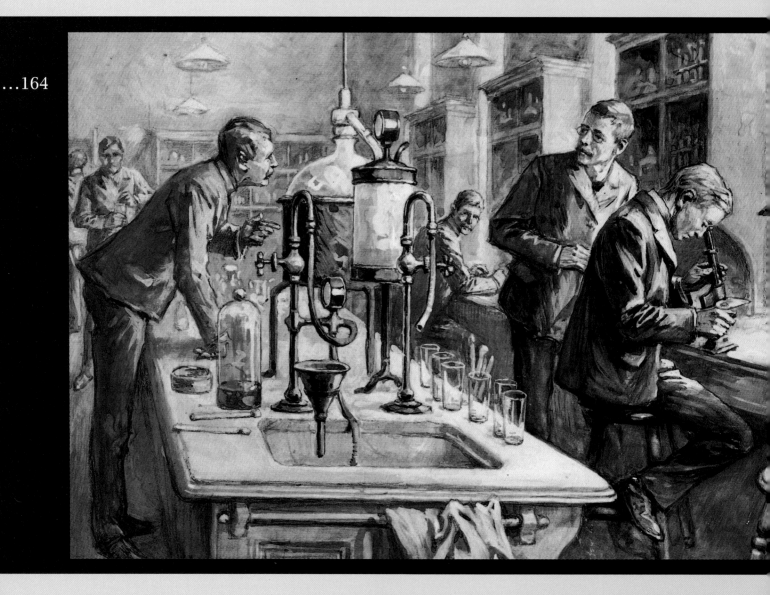

We have seen how the nineteenth and the early years of the twentieth century provided several of the means of achieving victory in the fight against infection, through the sciences of bacteriology, which characterized more and more organisms responsible for individual diseases, and immunology, which showed how the host responded to pathogens and enabled therapy to be devised to make best use of this response. It is now known that phagocytosis is the principal defence mechanism against bacteria, and so when the blood is deficient in normal white cells (as in some diseases of the bone marrow) the body falls prey to infections of all kinds. Phagocytosis probably removes the bacteria that have been made ineffective by antibodies, which are not often directly lethal. Other components in the serum necessary for the function of antibodies are 'complement' and 'opsonin', a group of substances discovered by Sir Almroth Edward Wright (1861–1947) which are probably antibodies that facilitate phagocytosis.

The serum of a healthy adult will contain very many different antibodies, each specific for a single disease: thus the antibodies of diphtheria will not give protection against tetanus. Antibodies are all proteins of the gamma-globulin group; all have a molecular weight of 160,000 to 1,00,000 and are identical chemically, so the differences which confer disease-specificity are very small. They are all produced by cells in the bone marrow and lymph nodes. The Australian Sir Frank Macfarlane Burnet (1899–1985) has remarked on the paradox that the self-same cells in the body which destroy worn-out cells (like

> The principle of transmission of disease by insects, suggested centuries earlier by the Indian Susruta, was soon applied to investigation of other disorders.

red blood cells) without the production of antibodies also get rid of foreign organisms with antibody production. This tolerance to one's own proteins is a learned reaction, acquired in the foetus before birth; injection of an antigen into a foetus in utero produces a lifelong tolerance to the antigen. Conversely, it is today believed that in certain diseases previously of unknown aetiology, the body loses its tolerance to a particular tissue, which is therefore damaged by immune processes. Today immunology has a bearing on still other aspects of medicine, including cancer treatment and spare-part surgery (because grafted donor tissues and organs tend to be rejected by the immune responses of the healthy body).

165...

Two further fields of achievement against infections have been the recognition of the role played by insects in the transmission of disease and the development of the science of virology.

Sir Patrick Manson (1844–1922), the 'father of modern tropic medicine', brought the existence of insect vectors (transmitters) to the attention of the medical world with a paper in 1877 in the *Medical Report of the Imperial Maritime Customs, China* in which he showed that a minute parasitic worm found in the human bloodstream – the cause of elephantiasis – was transmitted to man by the mosquito *Culex fatigans*, in which it developed. The principle of transmission of disease by insects, suggested many centuries earlier in the writings of the great Indian surgeon, Susruta, was soon applied to the investigation of other disorders. In 1882 Carlos Juan Finlay (1833–1915) reported evidence of the part played by the mosquito *Aëdes aegypti* in the spread of yellow fever in Cuba, and this was proved by Walter Reed and others in 1900. The causative agent of malaria, a protozoal plasmodium, was first seen by Charles Louis Alphonse Laveran (1845–1922) of Algiers in 1880, and in 1898 Sir Ronald Ross (1857–1932) found the parasite in the stomach of the Anopheles mosquito after it had fed on the blood of malarial patients, thus proving that the insect was responsible for the transmission of the disease. This knowledge was at once applied to the prevention of the disease; Sir Ronald Ross won a Nobel prize for his work in 1902 and Alphonse Laveran in 1907.

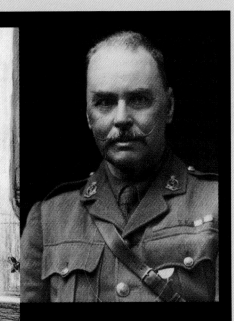

Above: Sir Ronald Ross, who won the Nobel prize in 1902 for his work on malaria.

Left: the laboratory of the Liverpool School of Tropical Medicine, 1899. On the left is Surgeon Major (later Sir) Ronald Ross. He is speaking to C S (later Sir Charles) Sherrington, then Holt Professor of Physiology. Rupert (later Sir) Rupert Boyce, the first dean of the school, is examining a slide on the right.

A new type of micro-organism was first recognized early in the twentieth century – *Rickettsia*, which are intermediate between bacteria and viruses in their size and characteristics. Charles Nicolle (1866–1936) showed in 1910 that the agent of infection of typhus fever was the body louse. This terrible epidemic disease was given one of its first accurate descriptions in 1530 by Fracastoro, the author of *Syphilis*, who at the same time set out the modern doctrine of the specific characters and infectious nature of fevers. The organism responsible for typhus remained unidentified for over 350 years. In 1909 Howard Ricketts (1871–1910) demonstrated the cause of a related disease, Rocky Mountain spotted fever, by examining the blood from infected patients. He died of typhus in the following year. In 1916 Henrique da Rocha-Lima (1879–1945) at last identified the agent responsible for typhus, which he named *Rickettsia prowazeki*, after Ricketts and another victim, Prowazek.

For centuries the term virus signified a poison produced by living beings and causing infectious disease. Viruses have been identified in the last sixty years in large numbers in a way comparable to the bacteriological discoveries of the end of the nineteenth century. This recent success is the result of special laboratory methods and in particular the use of the electron microscope – which makes visible minute particles beyond the resolving power of the ordinary instrument – stimulated by a number of terrible twentieth-century epidemics. The most terrible of these was the great influenza pandemic of 1918 to 1919, which spread throughout Europe, Russia, North and South America, New Zealand, Australia, Africa, India, China and Japan, an estimated 21,000,000 people dying of the disease. The virus, which like all viruses passes through the finest filter (in contrast to bacteria), was transmitted to ferrets by Wilson Smith (1897–1965), C H Andrewes (1896–1988) and Sir Patrick Laidlaw (1881–1940) in 1933, and cultured on developing eggs by Burnet two years later. This was virus A, which was found in London; a second virus, influenza B, was isolated in 1940 by Thomas Francis (b. 1900) in New York.

The use of the electron microscope, with its vast powers of magnification, has revolutionized the study of viruses.

Encephalitis lethargica or 'sleepy sickness' accompanied influenza, appearing in 1917 and continuing until 1926, when it virtually disappeared. It produced drowsiness, fits and coma, and, if the patient recovered, a common sequel was a form of Parkinson's disease. Another virus disease of the nervous system is poliomyelitis. This was first described at the end of the eighteenth century, but its epidemic and infective nature was not recognized until the work of Oscar Medin (1890) and Wickman (1907). In 1909 Simon Flexner (1863–1946) and Paul A Lewis (1879–1929) succeeded in producing paralysis in monkeys with virus derived from infected nasal secretion. Later the properties of the virus were fully established and several different varieties emerged; and in 1954 Jonas Salk introduced his vaccine, made from killed virus grown on monkey kidney cells and given by injection. More recently the oral Sabin vaccine, based on attenuated virus, has come into general use. The vaccines provide real protection; it should be remembered that viruses – from that of the common cold to smallpox – are unaffected by antibiotics and virtually the sole defence against them is a good level of antibodies.

Despite Ehrlich's work, however, it was not until 1935, with the introduction of prontosil by Gerhard Domagk (1895–1964), that the era of modern chemotherapy could be said to have begun. Prontosil contained sulphanilamide, which had been synthesized as long before as 1908, and after Domagk several investigators worked out that the sulphonamide group in the compound was the effective part. In 1938 a new drug, sulphapyridine (M and B 693), was first used in the treatment of pneumonia, and since then this and

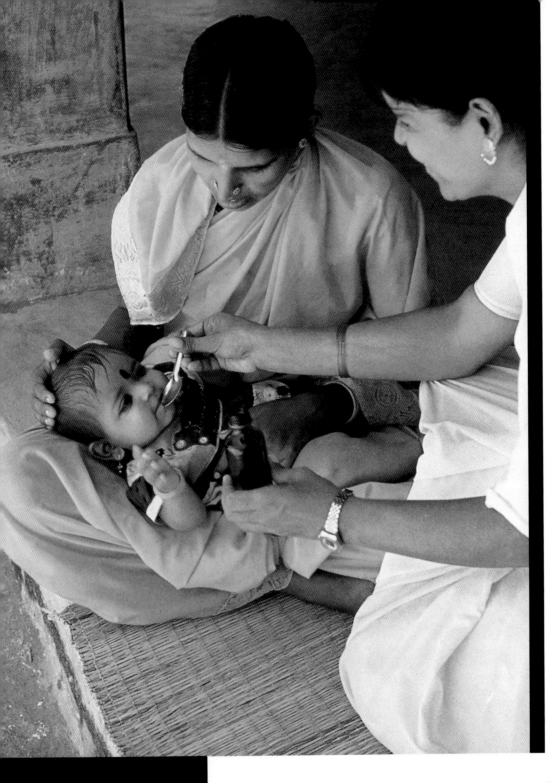

Above: in India, a nurse administers an oral vaccine against poliomyelitis, a viral disease of the nervous system.

many other sulphonamides have become an important and permanent part of the pharmacopoeia.

That many bacteria and fungi in the soil survive in the face of great competition for foodstuffs is a remarkable fact, and is due to their production of substances which spread into the surrounding soil and kill, or inhibit the growth of other species. This is the phenomenon of antibiosis and these substances are antibiotics. It was recognized for some time before Fleming's discovery of penicillin, for back in 1876 the Irish physicist John Tyndall (1820–92) had observed the selective bacteria-inhibiting action of Penicillium mould, while in the following year Pasteur and Joubert showed that airborne organisms inhibited anthrax.

Sir Alexander Fleming (1881–1955) made his first contribution to microbiology when he discovered lysozyme, which could dissolve living bacteria, in tears and egg white. His historic chance observation was made in 1928, when

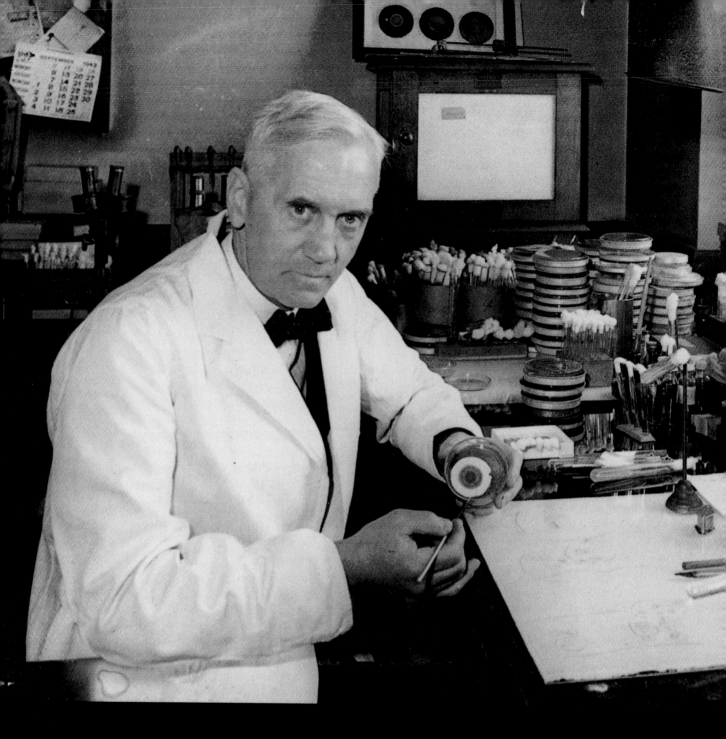

One of the greatest landmarks in the development of modern drugs was the discovery of penicillin by Sir Alexander Fleming in 1928, while studying a culture of staphylococci. Howard Florey and Ernst Chain continued the work some years later and penicillin was isolated in 1940.

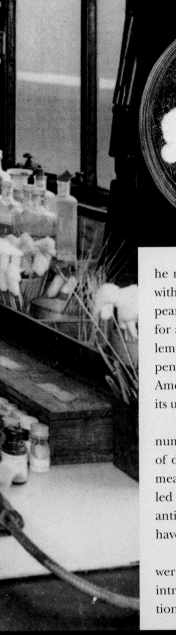

Left: the original culture plate of the fungus, *Penicillum notatum* made by Sir Alexander Fleming and rephotographed twenty-five years after his discovery in 1928.

Far left: Sir Alexander Fleming at work. Although Fleming discovered penicillin, he did not realise its full significance.

he noticed the contamination of a culture of staphylococci on an agar plate with the fungus *Penicillium notatum* caused colonies around the mould to disappear. Fleming continued his work at St Mary's Hospital, Paddington, London, for a while and published his observations in 1929. Investigation of the problem was pursued at Oxford by Sir Howard Florey and Ernst Chain, and penicillin was isolated in 1940. Within a few years it was being produced in America from cultures in vats of thousands of gallons of nutrient solution, and its use in the war greatly reduced Allied casualties.

Since the discovery of penicillin, there has been a vast increase in the number of antimicrobials available and today doctors have a bewildering array of drugs to choose from. The growth in the number of antibiotics does not mean that infections have been eradicated. The bacteria's ability to adapt has led to a rise in new infections by bacteria that no longer respond to traditional antibiotics such as MRSA (*Methicilin resistant staphylococcus aureus*). Newer drugs have been designed to overcome resistant organisms.

169...

Antibiotics can only treat bacterial infections and until recently there were no agents available to treat viral infections. In the mid-1980s acylovir was introduced, a drug with a specific action on herpes simplex and varicella infections. Subsequently manufacturers are developing a range of products to tackle other viral infections. Perhaps the greatest threat to modern man is the emergence of new life-threatening viruses for which there is no cure. Among this group is HIV (human immunodeficiency virus) and the more exotic viruses emerging from Africa, such as Ebola viruses. HIV is spread by bodily fluids and during unprotected sexual intercourse. The massive increase in HIV related illnesses and full-blown AIDS is as a result of the HIV virus damaging the immune response of the affected person.

The introduction of immunisation programmes in many countries was hailed as a major step forward in the management of infectious disease. The ultimate aim of vaccination is to provide immunity in the whole population and to reduce the adverse side-effects of the illness. In most developed countries measles, mumps and rubella, tuberculosis, and haemophilus influenza, diphtheria, tetanus and polio are all included in immunisation schedules. Immunisation alone will not prevent these infections occuring. Critics of mass immunisation programmes point to the dramatic fall in these conditions through good public health and hygiene measures.

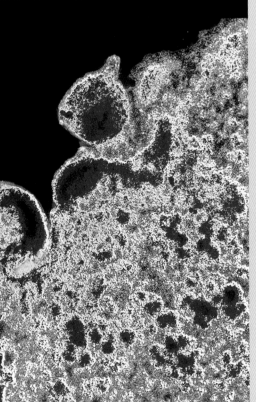

Left: false-colour transmission electron micrograph showing a single HIV virus particle magnified by 37,000 at 35 mm size.

X-RAYS AND OTHER METHODS OF DIAGNOSIS

It was a chance discovery by a German physicist that gave modern medicine one of its most powerful tools – X-rays. Wilhelm Konrad Roentgen (1845–1923) began studying electrical phenomena when he was professor of physics at the university of Würzburg. His experiments involved the passage of electricity through vacuum tubes; his momentous discovery occurred on the evening of 8 November 1895, when he noted that, while passing current through such a tube, a sheet of cardboard coated with barium platinocyanide was shining brightly in his unlit laboratory. He found that this fluorescence was a result of radiation coming from the tube. He called the radiation X-rays,

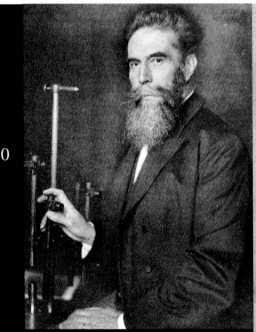

...170

Above: Wilhelm Konrad Roentgen. His discovery of X-rays was greeted with widespread enthusiasm.

Right: Roentgen's X-ray photograph of his wife's hand taken on 22 December 1895. Her ring appears as a deep black shadow.

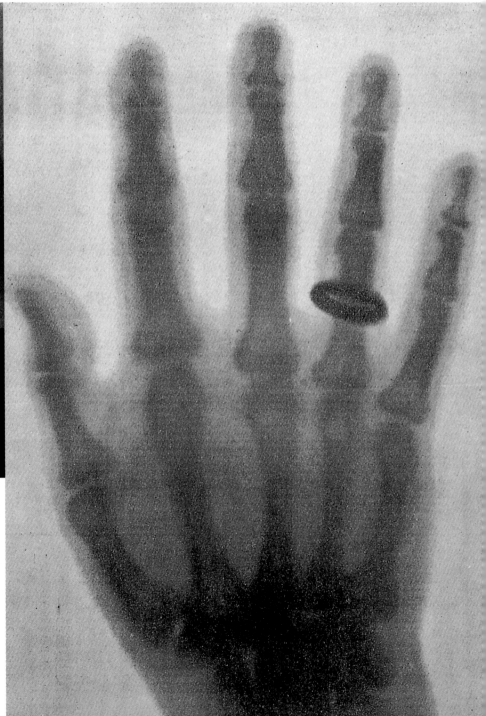

because of the unknown nature of the phenomenon; he soon found that the X-rays had the property of penetrating dense bodies opaque to light waves and giving an image on a photographic plate as well as on a fluorescent screen.

Roentgen then put solid objects between a Crookes tube and a wooden box in which he had placed a photographic plate, and discovered that an impression could be recorded on the plate, on which showed the form of each object. In another experiment, the physicist used his own hand: the bones were clearly shown on the plate, while the soft tissues were scarcely noticeable, as can be seen in his early photograph of his wife's hand, with a ring on the fourth finger. On 28 December 1895, Roentgen reported his sensational findings in his *Preliminary Communication to the President of the Physical-Medical Society of Würzburg*, fully aware of the implications of these mysterious rays for diagnosis. Within a few weeks his discovery had been greeted all over the world as one of the most important in medical history.

X-rays were used immediately in hospitals to diagnose fractures, bone diseases and foreign bodies. The first apparatus was primitive and emitted weak radiation; to obtain a radiograph it was necessary to allow an exposure time of nearly thirty minutes. It was soon noticed that X-rays caused unpleasant and slowly healing skin burns. The necessity of reducing the exposure time was at once recognized, and in 1913 this was achieved with the introduction of the heated cathode which emitted a greater quantity of electrons of higher energy than a cold cathode. During the First World War, ample use was found for the improved equipment, which required an exposure of a few seconds, in locating bullets and shell fragments.

Improvement has continued and today X-ray films require only a fraction of the exposure time and the pictures are very much clearer. Technical advances involve filters, diaphragms and more efficient fluorescent materials, on the one hand, and new investigative methods on the other. W B Cannon (1871–1945), while a medical student, introduced the use of bismuth – which is radio-opaque – for observing the intestines and stomachs of animals. Contrast radiography has developed from this, and now barium sulphate taken by mouth is used to outline the gastro-intestinal tract, while iodinated substances can be injected into veins to show the kidneys and into arteries to show the circulation in any part of the body, including the brain. The various body cavities can also be outlined by the injection of air. Tomography enables a plane section of any organ to be visualized.

The hands and exposed parts of the first radiologists suffered chronic and painful rashes and burns; many of these pioneers, ignorant of the powerful biological effect of X-rays, in fact died of skin cancer and leukaemia. Doctors began to use the new rays to treat skin diseases shortly after they were discovered, and then to treat skin cancer, and a few years later, when their powerful actions on germinal or rapidly dividing cells were known, to treat a wide range of malignant diseases. With lead shields and accurate dosimetry, radiotherapy became practical, although deep-seated lesions could not be dealt with satisfactorily at first because of the poor penetration of the rays and severe skin effects.

A chance discovery in 1895 led to the development of X-rays by the German physicist, Wilhelm Konrad Roentgen.

171...

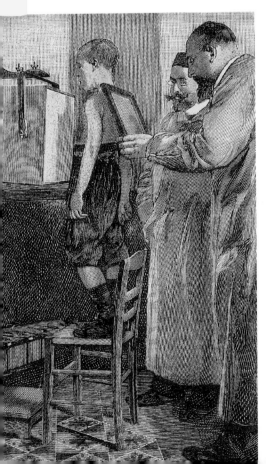

Left: a woodcut, circa 1900, showing the use of X-rays for the early diagnosis of tuberculosis.

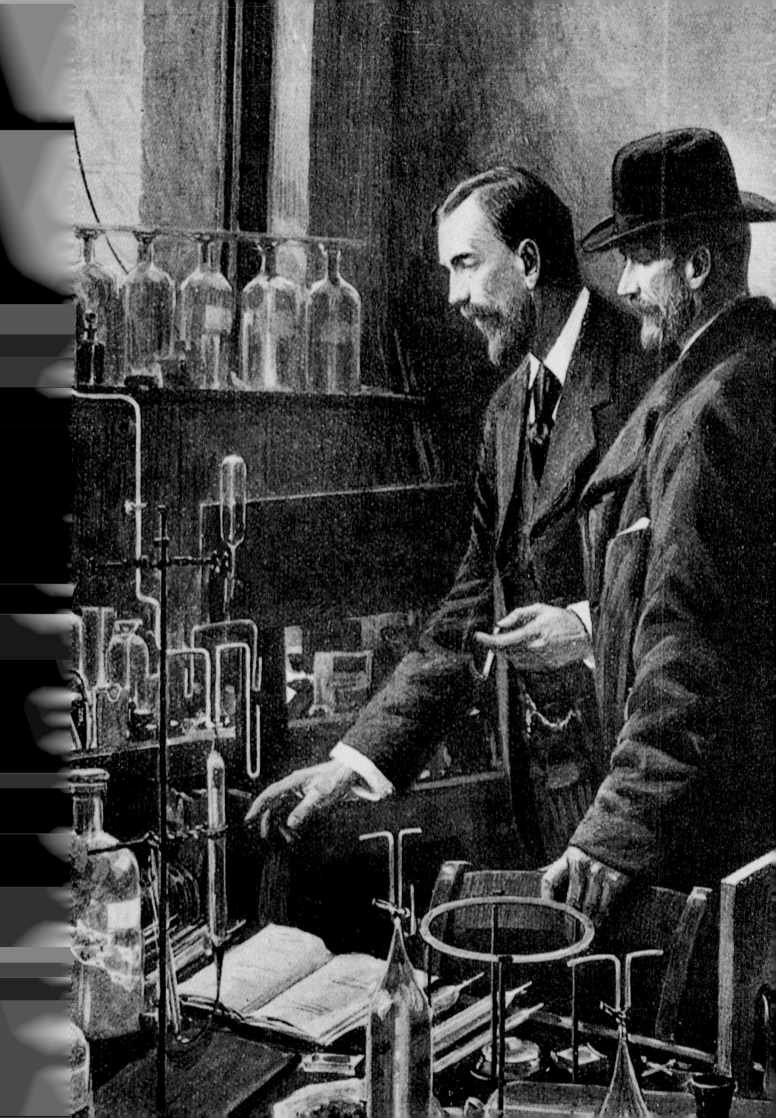

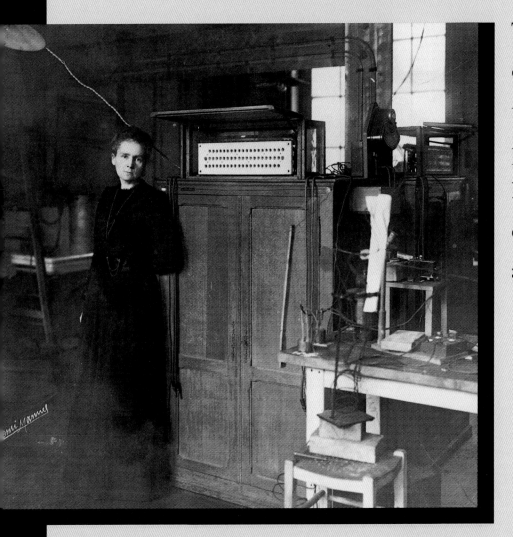

The development
of the therapeutic
uses of radium
paralleled that of
X-rays, whose
effects on tissues
are similar.

173...

Above: Marie Curie, photographed in her laboratory in 1910. She was a Nobel prizewinner in 1903 and 1911, the first person to be twice honoured.

Left: Pierre Curie with Sir William Ramsay.

Natural radioactivity was discovered in uranium salts by the great French physicist Henri Becquerel, Nobel prizewinner for 1903. Becquerel found that a photographic plate was blackened by the invisible rays emitted by uranium salts even when wrapped in a layer of black paper and of silver. In 1898 Pierre Curie and his assistant, later his wife, Maria Sklodovska, isolated polonium and discovered radium. Pierre purposely produced a burn on his arm with radium, which was soon found to be destructive to animal tissues and effective in the treatment of tumours. The Curies were awarded a Nobel prize in 1904. Like Roentgen, prizewinner in 1901, they refused to patent their discovery. When her husband died in 1906, Marie Curie succeeded to his chair of physics at the Sorbonne and in 1910 she isolated metallic radium

The major problem of radiotherapy was to reach the tumour with radiation strong enough to attack or even destroy it, while damaging the normal cells as little as possible. The first X-rays from low-voltage apparatus had limited therapeutic value because of skin damage. The first machine capable of emitting radiation which could reach comparatively deep-seated tumours, such as those of the breast, was of 250,000 volts. Before the Second World War more powerful machines were built, including some with voltages in the millions; in use these proved to be disappointing. After the war, radiotherapy entered a new phase thanks to electronic technology and isotope chemistry.

The development of the therapeutic uses of radium paralleled that of X-rays, whose effects on tissues are similar. In the form of radioactive needles and seeds, implanted into malignant tissue, it has found an important place in the treatment especially of tumours of the cervix, bladder and tongue.

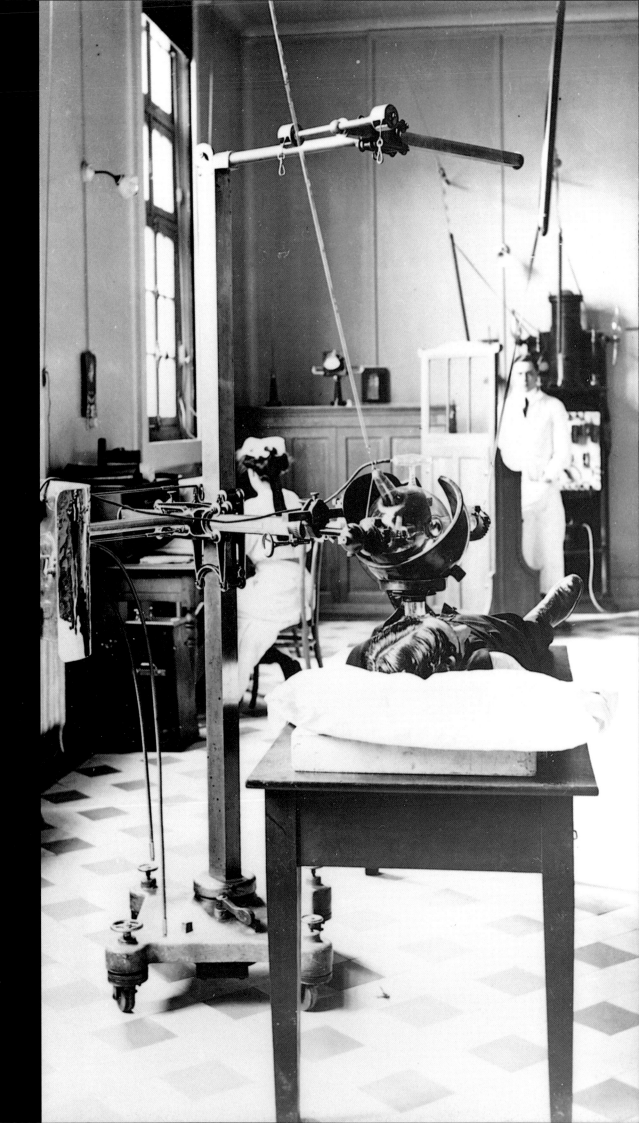

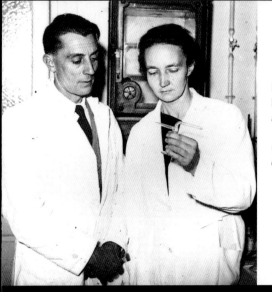

Left: Irène Curie and her husband Frédéric Joliot, Nobel prizewinners in 1935 for their work on artificial radioactivity.

Far left: a demonstration of radiotherapy at the Cochi Hospital in Paris in 1905.

Since the discovery in 1931 of artificial radioactivity by Irène Curie and her husband Frédéric Joliot, radioactive isotopes have found innumerable uses in medical research, diagnosis and treatment.

From the chemical viewpoint, radioactive isotopes are indistinguishable from stable isotopes of the same atomic number, but they differ in their emission of alpha and beta particles (helium nuclei and electrons) and gamma rays (X-rays). Their presence is thus detectable with appropriate apparatus and they can take part in the body in the same processes as their stable counterparts.

The use of minute quantities of isotopes as tracers to outline metabolic pathways in the body began with the work of Georg von Hevesy, and has led to the concept of 'the dynamic state of body constituents' (whereby all the molecules of the tissues are in a constant state of flux), as well as detailed knowledge of the metabolism of fats, carbohydrates, proteins and electrolytes. Substances such as iron, hormones or drugs can be 'labelled' and their progress followed as they travel through the body. Information about the growth and multiplication of cells can be obtained by the use of nucleic acid precursors containing radioactive hydrogen or carbon.

175...

Since the discovery in 1931 of artificial radioactivity, radioactive isotopes have found innumerable uses in medical research, diagnosis and treatment.

In diagnosis, isotopes are used to measure abnormal activity of various parts of the body. Radioactive iodine is taken up by the thyroid, and after a patient has drunk a small quantity of this substance the gland can be scanned for uptake. Other radioactive substances are concentrated in tumours, and this fact is of particular value in the localization of brain tumours. Red blood cells can be tagged and their life span in the body calculated in some cases of anaemia. Abnormal kidney blood flow can be investigated by the excretion of a labelled compound. These and many other uses indicate the importance of isotopes as diagnostic tools.

From the point of view of therapy, the chief use of an isotope is that of iodine in cases where the thyroid gland is overactive. Here a much larger quantity is used than in diagnosis; the isotope accumulates in the thyroid and the rays it emits damage the hormone-producing cells. As has been mentioned, isotopes have supplanted high-voltage X-rays: telecobalt therapy utilizes the emission from an unstable form of cobalt to irradiate deep tumours intensely for a short period. This technique has the advantage of reducing radiation damage to neighbouring tissues.

Another therapeutic use of cell-damaging ionizing radiation is in suppressing the immune mechanisms of the body and so enabling grafts of foreign tissue to be accepted. Since antibody production will cause rejection of tissue from any other individual (except an identical twin) irradiation of the whole body combined with cortisone and other drugs which counter the immune response is at present essential to the success of spare-part surgery.

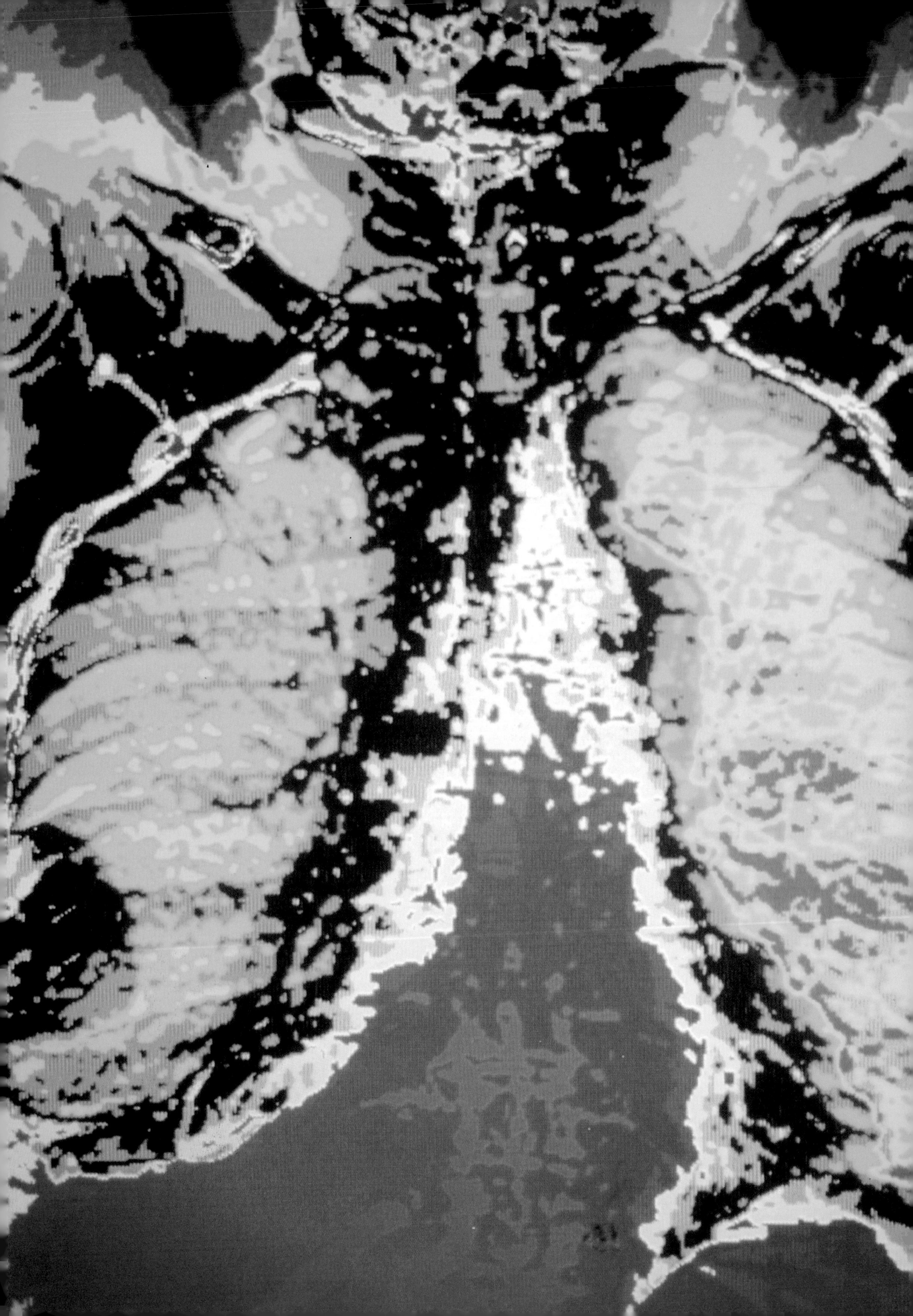

X-rays and other radiographic and imaging techniques now form an important part of the doctor's armoury when diagnosing disease. Modern X-ray techniques allow for safer exposure to lower levels of radiation. New techniques which do not require major intrusion into the body have been developed over the past twenty years. It is now possible to see inside the abdomen using ultrasound scanning. So successful is this technique that it is now used to screen pregnant women for birth defects.

CAT (computerised axial tomography) scanning was introduced in 1975, A CT scan takes several pictures of the body at different points around the area being filmed, rather like slices through a loaf of bread. It is able to show more detail of the inner organs than a standard X-ray. The picture produced is a result of a computer analysis of the multiple pictures that have been taken.

It is possible that in certain conditions even CT scanning is now being superseded by MRI (magnetic resonance imaging), which was developed in the late 1970s and introduced for diagnostic purposes in 1983, and which is able to produce sophisticated images of the internal organ systems. MRI scans are particularly useful for showing soft tissue injuries within the spine, such as a prolapsed disc, or a torn cartilage within a knee joint. Patients having CT and MRI scans have to lie still, within the scanner, for up to thirty minutes, but the procedure is painfree.

CAT scanning, introduced in 1975, may well be superceded by MRI imaging methods.

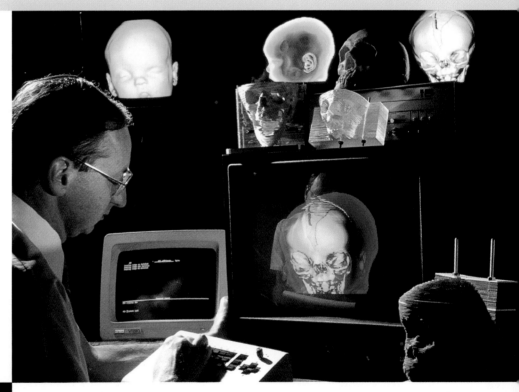

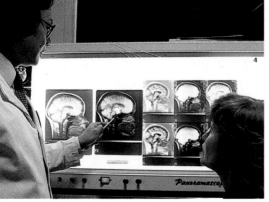

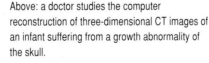

Above: a doctor studies the computer reconstruction of three-dimensional CT images of an infant suffering from a growth abnormality of the skull.

Left: two scientists examine MRI images of the human brain.

Far left: a CT scan showing a posterior view of a cancerous lung. The light blue areas in the right lung indicate the cancerous formations.

NERVOUS AND MENTAL DISEASES

What we know to be mental illness belonged, for early man, to the sphere of the supernatural, the result of possession of the victim by evil spirits. Treatmemt involved the use of amulets and charms imbued with magical powers. However, through the centuries, the vehicles of faith and magic in healing gradually changed from material to ritual, from precious objects to secret words and formulae and mystical numbers, while the civilized world endowed its religions with therapeutic powers.

For a long period after the rise of Christianity, spiritual treatment, or faith-healing, and the charm-laden medicine of folklore coexisted and were used alike to help the mentally ill. But as the Church became more powerful and authoritarian, unorthodoxy was suppressed and folk remedies were stigmatized as witchcraft, as indeed were manifestations of psychiatric illness. It was only with the Renaissance, and the victory of knowledge over supersitition, that a more rational attitude came about.

The first attempts to classify psychiatric disease were made in the eighteenth century, and, at the same time, restraint, starvation, close confinement and other violent methods began to be supplanted by more humane treatment. An important name is that of William Cullen (1710–90), the spiritual head of the sect of 'neuropathlogists' and a great influence for many years. By asserting that 'life, so far as it is corporeal, consists in the excitement of the nervous system and especially of the brain, which unites the different parts, and forms them into a whole', he paved the way for modern neurophysiology and the work of Pavlov and Sherrington.

At this time, doctors began systematically to differentiate and classify psychiatric diseases in the same way as physical complaints. Violent methods gave way to therapy designed for helpless patients in need of care, and this change of attitude on the part of physicians and society accompanied the transformation of 'mad-houses' into 'asylums', well-regulated hospitals where the insane might be nursed rather than filthy prisons where they could be left to die. This movement began in Italy with Vincenzo Chiarugi in 1744 and in England it was initiated by William Tuke, a Quaker tea merchant who founded a retreat at York in 1794. In France, Philippe Pinel was the first to apply to the insane the humanitarian principles of the revolutionaries. Appointed physician to the asylum at Bicêtre in 1793, he released his fettered charges and showed, with his superior practical sense, that insane people, like any other sick human beings, could be treated by physicians without loss of dignity. He stated that moral persuasion was better than intimidation and force, and that a strong personality on the part of the physician was the greatest factor in success. He put great store in good administration, and having reformed the Bicêtre he moved to the

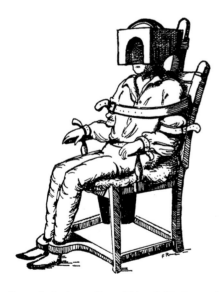

Above: the barbarous 'tranquillizing chair' advocated by the American, Benjamin Rush.

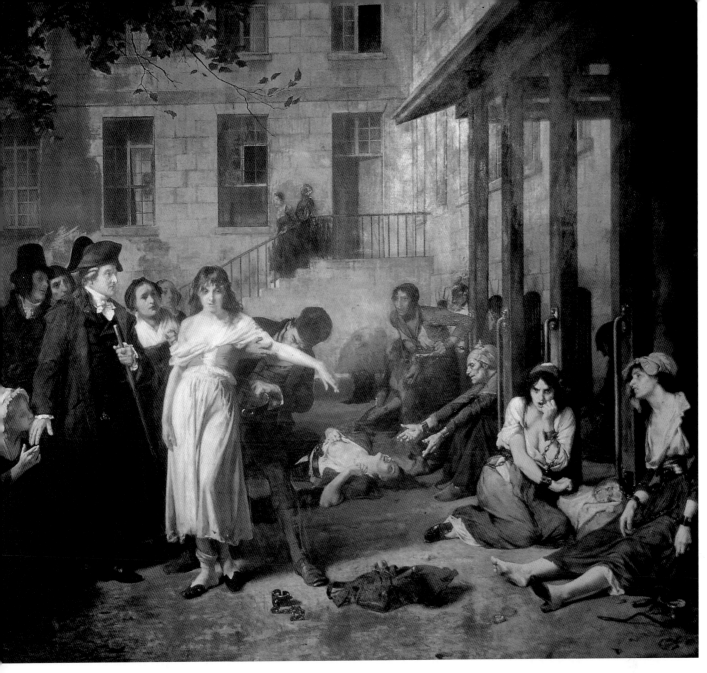

Above: Philippe Pinel ordering the chains to be removed from the patients at the Salpêtrière in Paris in 1795.

Salpêtrière where by careful observation and note-taking he gradually built up a method of clinical psychiatry.

In the early nineteenth century, psychiatry and neurology were developing in a number of other ways. Mesmerism, despite being surrounded at first by spectacular showmanship, was to provide a powerful psychotherapeutic tool. Phrenology, whereby moral and intellectual qualities were supposedly ascertainable from a study of the external configuration of the skull, was initiated by Franz Joseph Gall (1758–1828) and elaborated to extreme length by his followers; its value was in showing for the first time that different regions of the brain might serve specific purposes, and from it developed the seminal concept of cerebral localization. Before long, the great physiologist Marie Jean Pierre Flourens (1794–1867) sited sensation and will in the cerebrum and showed that the cerebellum was responsible for co-ordination of movement and the medulla for respiration. Clinical observation continued to improve, and clear pictures of disease entities emerged; a classic is the 1817 essay of the Hoxton general practitioner and freethinker James Parkinson (1755–1824) on 'shaking palsy' (Parkinson's disease).

Experimental results continued to clarify neuro-physiology. Charles Bell (1774–1842) and François Magendie (1783–1855) showed that the anterior and posterior roots of the nerves coming from the spinal cord were functionally distinct, and were concerned respectively with sensibility and movement, and Marshall Hall (1790–1857) expounded the idea of the reflex arc.

The advance of knowledge in this field in the mid-nineteenth century accompanied improved diagnosis, for in no other branch of medicine as in neurology can a disease state be related to a disturbance in part of the nervous system. Brown-Séquard threw light on the sensory and motor functions of the spinal cord, Claude Bernard on the sympathetic nerves, and Paul Broca (1824–80) on the association of speech disturbance (aphasia) with damage to a small part of the left cerebral hemisphere. The synthesis was achieved by Jean-Martin Charcot (1825–93), under whom the Salpêtrière in Paris became the centre of neurology. Charcot's reputation and genius lay in his universal approach, for he was the first to use regional criteria (acknowledging the concept that different parts of the nervous system have different functions) and pathological criteria in diagnosis. He described exactly such conditions as tabes dorsalis, motor neurone disease and multiple sclerosis, and he produced a mas-

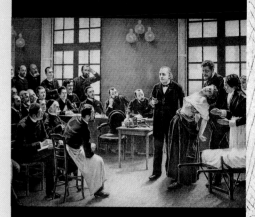

Above: Jean-Martin Charcot demonstrating the nature of hysteria at the Salpêtrière, circa 1885.

terly account of hysteria and hypnotic states, distinguished from organic disturbances by careful evaluation of symptoms and physical signs. By defining hysteria and hypnosis, which the Salpêtrière school thought to be identical, Charcot transformed these subjects from a spectacle into a science.

In the 1880s, the Nancy school under Hippolyte Bernheim (1840–1919) argued against Charcot's thesis that a hysterical disposition occurred only in certain patients, and showed that hypnotism was an intensification of normal suggestion. This idea was widely adopted in the closing years of the century, and hypnotism came to be used in the treatment of neuroses and alcoholism. Dominated by Charcot and Bernheim, French psychiatry continued to concern itself mainly with neuroses, and this emphasis was of great importance as it led to the discovery of psychoanalysis. Here Pierre Janet (1859–1947) should be mentioned; he formulated a concept of mental automatism in hysteria and recognized hysterical dissociation and the existence of unconscious factors.

Meanwhile, in Germany, neurological and psychiatric illnesses were closely studied in the nineteenth century. But the approach was self-limiting in that it described and pigeonholed diseases, but ignored the causes.

Sigmund Freud (1856–1939) threw light on the unconscious factors outlined by Janet. He studied neuroanatomy and neuropathology in Vienna and in 1855 went to the Salpêtrière. Modern psychoanalytic methods can be said to have been initiated by Freud in the following year, when he returned to Vienna after working with Charcot on hypnosis as a treatment for hysterical patients. He found that this method was not always effective since only some of his patients could be hypnotized, and even those who could be were not often helped. Together with Josef Breuer (1842–1925), he evolved a method through which patients could discuss their emotional problems by free association, whereby 'powerful emotional drives swept the uncontrolled thoughts in the direction of psychic conflict'.

From his observations of patients under these conditions Freud found that forgotten or painful memories could often be related to traumatic sexual experiences in childhood; he concluded that hysteria resulted from childhood seduction and obsessional neurosis from guilt of active participation in such an event. He then elaborated his hypothesis of unconscious motivation, repression and resistance (whereby an experience becomes and is maintained unconscious) and the causation of neurosis. This resulted from repression of painful memories that were 'incompatible with the other dominant tendencies of the personality'.

Above: Sigmund Freud, left, photographed with Carl Gustav Jung at Clark University in 1909.

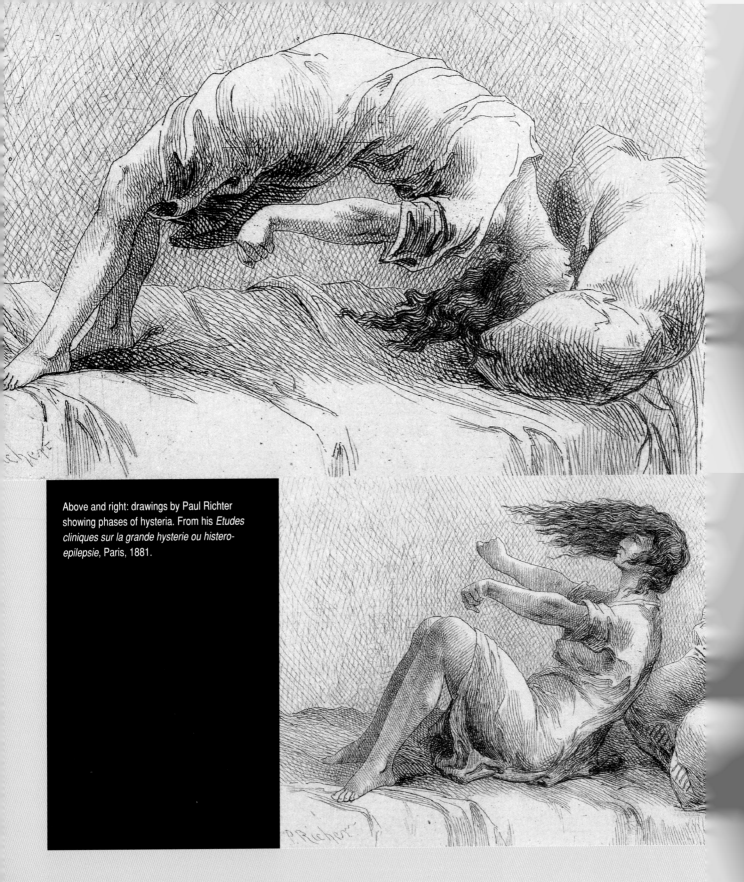

Above and right: drawings by Paul Richter showing phases of hysteria. From his *Etudes cliniques sur la grande hysterie ou histero-epilepsie*, Paris, 1881.

Together with Josef Breuer, Freud
evolved a method whereby patients could
discuss their emotional problems
by free association.

However, Freud soon realised that childhood seduction could only occasionally be implicated. Slips of the tongue and dreams were unconsciously motivated in many cases, and other processes might be at work. Freud thus elaborated the concepts of infantile sexuality and the Oedipus complex to explain imagined seduction by the parent of the opposite sex. Briefly, the infant in growing up was thought to go through three phases in which the main desires were satisfied by the mouth, the anus and the genitalia. Pre-genital sexuality ended at the age of three, but conflicts sooner or later might cause fixation at a regression to an earlier phase. At three, boys wanted the attention of their mother and resented their father – the Oedipus complex. Girls would later develop an Electra complex whereby they would desire their father and reject their mother, and these complexes were regarded as the source of anxiety, whereby libido was dammed up and not directed into the proper channels of adult sexuality and mature behaviour.

About this time, Freud classified mental functions into conscious, preconscious and unconscious (the last being actively repressed and not able voluntarily to be recognized), and later he developed his theories of the ego (the conscious being), the superego (parental and social 'conscience') and the id (the source of mental energy, desires and libido). The id is the only mind of the newborn child and gradually becomes overshadowed by the ego and the superego; its aims remain, however, and repression, inhibition and sublimation of these leads respectively to neurosis, sexual deviation and artistic creativity.

Freud's final contribution was to attribute the origin of all anxiety to separation from the mother, which resulted in unknown internal danger. His various followers have changed his basic theories in a number of ways and have all underplayed the sexual theme on which he put so much emphasis. Carl Gustav Jung (1875–1961) introduced the idea of archetypes and the collective unconscious, a repository of experiences belonging to the race, and the concept of introversion and extroversion. Alfred Adler (1870–1937) suggested that the inferiority complex was the most important driving factor in the armoury of the libido. Otto Rank (1884–1939), taking the childhood theme to extremes, postulated that anxiety began in the womb at the time of birth, when the child is subjected to a temporary asphyxia.

From the second half of the nineteenth century, neurology was advanced on the one hand by anatomy and microscopy, especially in Germany, and on the other by physiological discoveries. Histological methods revealed the fine structure of the nervous system and, at the same time morbid anatomy gave precise pathological meaning to a variety of nervous diseases. On the neurophysiological front advantage was taken of graphic methods of recording and electrical apparatus to study nervous tissues. The electrical excitability of nerve and muscle had long been known; Gustav Fritsch (1838–97) and Eduard Hitzig (1838–1907) were the first to show (in 1870) that excitation of particular areas of the cerebral cortex could produce contraction of localized groups of muscles. Many other investigators developed knowledge of cerebral localization, vital to diagnosis and treatment, and with the discovery by Caton of Birmingham of the intrinsic electrical activity of the brain, the development of the electro-encephalograph (EEG) was foreshadowed.

Neurophysiology in England was crowned at the end of the century by the work of Charles Sherrington (1861–1952), who developed the views of Bell and Magendie on spinal activity and in *The Integrative Action of the Nervous System* produced the classic work on the nature of reflexes, the foundation of modern ideas of the functioning of the brain and spinal cord. Meanwhile, clinical neu-

> At three, boys wanted the attention of their mother and resented their father – the Oedipus complex. Girls would later develop the Electra complex.

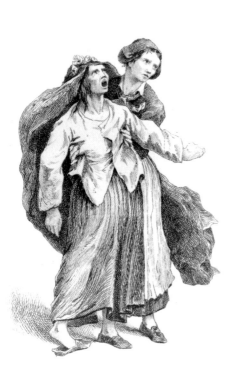

Above: Epilepsy – agitation and partial spasm. A drawing by Paul Richter from his *Etudes cliniques sur la grande hystérie ou histero-epilepsie*, Paris, 1881.

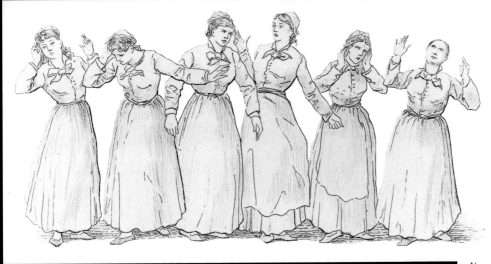

Above: Catalepsy, a drawing by Paul Richter from his *Etudes cliniques sur la grande hysterie ou histero-epilepsie*, Paris, 1881. Catalepsy is marked by a state of almost complete insensibility. This drawing shows six women in cataleptic states brought on by an unexpected loud noise.

rologists in France and Germany widened the frontiers of knowledge by describing many previously unrecognized forms of nervous disease. It was in England, however, that modern neurology began with the work of John Hughlings Jackson (1835–1911), who, influenced by Brown-Séquard, came to the National Hospital for the Paralysed and Epileptic in London soon after its foundation in 1860. He defined the nervous system as an organ arranged and working at different levels of evolution, and he distinguished between 'discharging' and 'destroying' lesions, the effect of the former being the epileptic fit and that of the latter paralysis. In both cases one part of the body (hand, face or foot) might be principally affected, and Jackson described the convul-

183...

sion as 'the mobile counterpart' of the stroke. He stated that dissolution of nervous function always progressed from the most voluntary, most specialized and most differentiated, to the most automatic, least specialized and least differentiated – paralysis, aphasia and dementia all obeyed this law.

> Freud taught that the roots of many mental conditons should be sought in the experiences and problems of the patient.

In the twentieth century, neurology and psychiatry have gained from developments in new methods of research and discoveries in different fields, which tend to fertilize each other. Thus biochemistry has revealed not only the existence and identity of chemical transmitters in the nervous system but also provides tests for the diagnosis of many diseases and has given a possible clue to the nature of schizophrenia. Advances in pharmacology on the one hand have given the scientist tools to investigate nervous functions and on the other hand effective treatment for such conditions as epilepsy, Parkinsonism and myasthenia gravis. Psychiatric treatment has been revolutionized by psychotropic drugs (like phenothiazines and mono-amine oxidase inhibitors) which have powerful effects on mental disturbances. The introduction of lithium-based products for treatment of manic-depressive illness, and depot injections of phenothiazines (drugs injected into the body which last for up to a month at a time) have helped to control the more serious mental illnesses. Recent advances in the treatment of depression include SSRI (serotonin re-uptake inhibitor) drugs, such as Prozac. These new anti-depressants work on elevating levels of the chemical serotonin in the brain, which is thought to be low in people suffering from depression.

The electron microscope is now revealing new facts. Radiology and isotope chemistry enable the neurologist to confirm his diagnosis by outlining the cerebral blood vessels (arteriography) and ventricles (pneumoencephalography and ventriculography) and scanning the brain for an area of radioactivity indicating isotope uptake by a tumour.

Neurosurgery has benefited particularly from advances in anaesthesia. The American, Harvey Cushing (1864–1939) extended the scope of the field beyond brain tumours, which he was the first to classify in a systematic and comprehensive manner according to prognostic and clinical criteria. Thanks to Cushing, neurosurgery now provides treatment for brain and spinal tumours, head injury, hydrocephalus and some cases of epilepsy and intractable pain, and more recently developments in neuroanatomy and physiology have enabled a successful surgical attack to be made on Parkinson's disease. Today's modern neurological units can also ligate bleeding blood vessels called aneurysms, which may cause strokes or even death. Experimental work on the implantation of fetal tissue into the brains of Parkinsonian patients has shown much promise. Stereo-tactic surgery, the insertion of fine probes into the brain which can destroy abnormal areas of tissue has been much enhanced by the advent of modern X-ray techniques such as CT scanners and MRI imaging which help to locate abnormalities more accurately.

Psychiatry has seen two revolutions – the psychoanalytical and the pharmacological – during the twentieth century.

The physiology of the nervous system is now well understood at the cellular level. Exploration of the nature of the nerve impulse began with the work of Keith Lucas (1879–1916) and continued with Lord Adrian (1889–1977) and others, using valve amplifiers and cathode ray tubes, and micro-methods have enabled electrical recordings to be made from individual nerve fibres and brain cells. Information continues to be gained about the activity of the brain as a whole. Sherrington apart, the most important name in this field is that of Ivan Petrovich Pavlov (1849–1936), much of whose work on conditioned reflexes was carried out at the end of the last century. He showed that frequent repetition of specific stimuli could produce reflexes bearing no direct relationship to the stimulus; thus bell-ringing, after having been sufficiently associated with the exhibition of food, could produce in dogs a flow of gastric juice even in the absence of food. Pavlov contrasted ordinary reflexes, which were momentary and transitory, with conditioned reflexes, which became gradually reinforced to become chronic manifestations. From his physiological findings

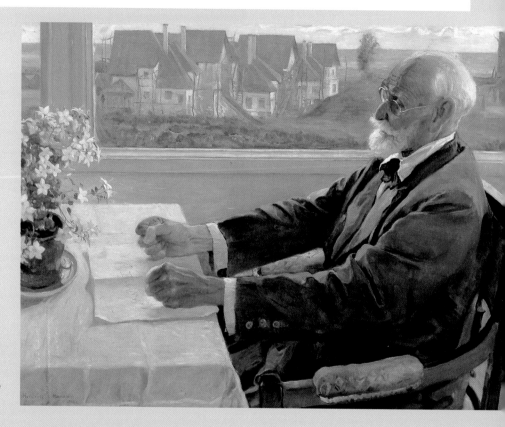

Right: Ivan Petrovich Pavlov, in 1934. Pavlov achieved widespread fame through his work on the conditioned reflex.

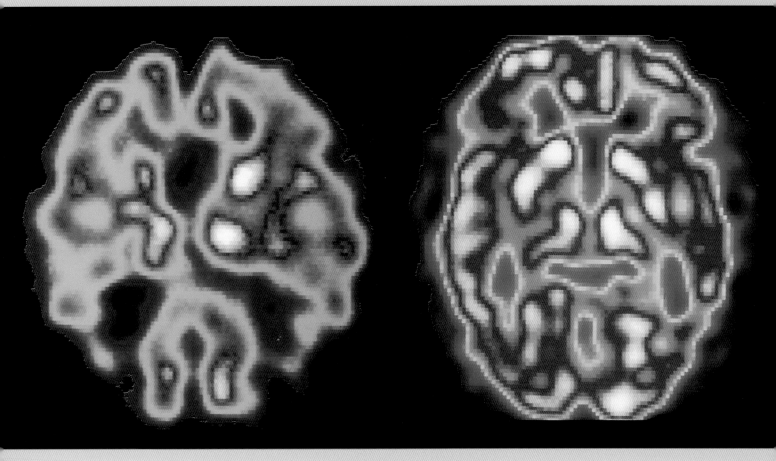

Above: Positive emission tomography (PET) scans of the human brain. The image on the left shows the brain of a patient suffering from Altzheimer's disease; the image on the right shows a normal brain. Normal brain metabolic activity produces a roughly symmetrical pattern in the yellow areas of the left and right cerebral hemispheres. The patchy appearance of the scan of the Altzheimer's patient indicates degeneration of the brain tissue.

he turned to psychiatry; having produced artificial neuroses in dogs by presenting two similar conditioning stimuli, he postulated that hysteria was the result of conflicting, overwhelmingly strong or weak repetitive stimuli impinging on the balanced mechanism of conditioning. Animals could be reconditioned back to normal, which suggested a therapy for neurotic patients. This turned out not to be very effective in the long run, but Pavlovian theory has been vindicated in human physiology, and at the present time, when doubt is being cast on fine cerebral localization of function, a holistic approach to the workings of the nervous system is of great value.

In contrast to neurology, where knowledge accrues little by little, psychiatry, having been overwhelmed by two revolutions – the psychoanalytical and pharmacological – in the present century, is today in a state of flux. As ever, there are two fundamental approaches to diagnosis and therapy, the psychological and the organic, but if there is a present-day trend it is to attempt to link these and to correlate in treatment psychoanalysis, modern drugs and assessment of the mentally sick individual in the background of his own environment. However, the problems to be resolved by modern psychiatry are not just those of the overtly ill mental patient. Psychosomatic diseases, physical states brought on by emotional conflict or stress, are now being recognized more and more. Besides, human existence must be seen in a psychological perspective, and psychiatric ideas thus impinge on all aspects of everyday life. For this reason the branches of child psychology and industrial psychology have developed and psychiatric social help is available to the community: contemporary psychiatry entails not only the modernization of mental hospitals and hospital treatment but also the evolution of altogether new and different systems of care for patients.

MEDICINE
PAST AND FUTURE

What is the value of medical history at the present time? What is the usefulness of a knowledge of medicine of the past to people of today? Before answering these questions it must be said that medical history remains largely separated from medical practice: medical historians are more often historians rather than practising doctors, and the training of most medical students, in Europe and America, generally ignores all but the most superficial excursions into the subject. Too often the new doctor leaves medical school in total ignorance of the evolution of his art and science, contemptuous of the mistakes of earlier generations of physicians and surgeons and at the same time half-blinded to new developments in medicine. To laymen, medical history must often seem of even less relevance to the present or the future.

Yet the inescapable truth – and the value of medical history is to remind one of it – is that today's medicine is something that has been built up over the centuries, succeeding eras seeing more or less important additions to the cor-

Right: the first stage in the preparation of 'artificial' skin. Using a tool known as a credo, a scientist separates the outer epidermis from the dermis in a small piece of fresh human skin. Later, cells of the epidermis are separated in a centrifuge and 'sown' on to a fragment of human dermis. After a few days, the result is an enlarged section of reconstituted skin.

Below: a researcher using a surgical simulator to practise eye surgery.

...186 Modern medicine is something that has been built up over the centuries, succeeding eras seeing more or less important additions to the corpus of medical knowledge and practice.

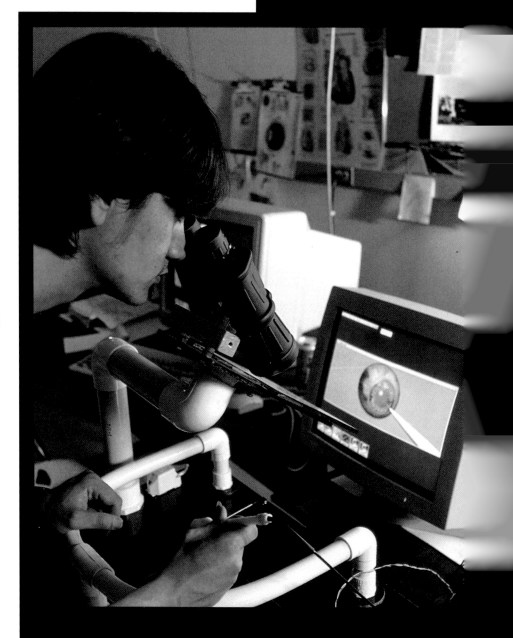

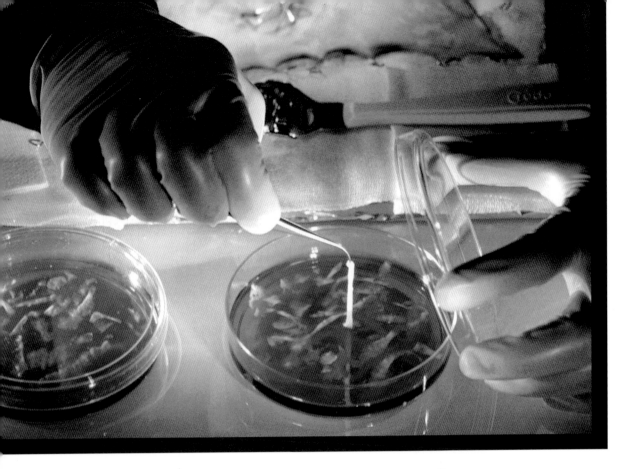

pus of medical knowledge and practice. The significance of many past discoveries to the present time has been pointed out in this book. The humane and yet reserved doctor is the descendant on one hand of Hippocrates and Sydenham, and on the other, of the Aesculapian priests. His ability to diagnose disease starts with his taking a history from the patient: again, this is something that stems from the ancients, from Hippocrates and Galen, and it is something which has nothing to do with scientific method. His clinical diagnostic methods, however, do belong to the age of science, and are the development of systems worked out in the eighteenth and nineteenth centuries by such people as Auenbrugger, Laënnec, and the Parisian and Queen Square neurologists. Already in the late twentieth century many of these procedures have become old-fashioned and supplanted by more modern techniques. Thus a very elaborate examination of the chest by the traditional practice of 'inspection, palpation, percussion and auscultation' is partly bypassed, because an equivalent or even a greater amount of information about the state of the lungs can be obtained very simply by X-raying the patient. New methods of pathological and chemical diagnosis have evolved, more rationally and less empirically based than the mediaeval practice of urinoscopy but occupying nevertheless an equivalent position in medical science. In due course the innovations of today will be themselves largely succeeded, a number surviving as valuable incorporations into the evolving mass of medicine.

Medicine is still a mixture of art, developing the skills to deal with people, and science, using the latest technological advances to enhance patient care.

The rapid advances made by scientific discovery mean that people are now living longer, but also that health services are having to deal with greater numbers of 'chronic illnesses'. This leads to new dilemmas for society. Which conditions can be treated? Are there sufficient resources to meet all the health needs of a developed society? Can people afford the health care they demand?

What of the future? Despite the improvements in health care, as a result of improved public health new challenges exist. The increasing number of elderly patients require more expensive treatments. Operations which thirty years ago

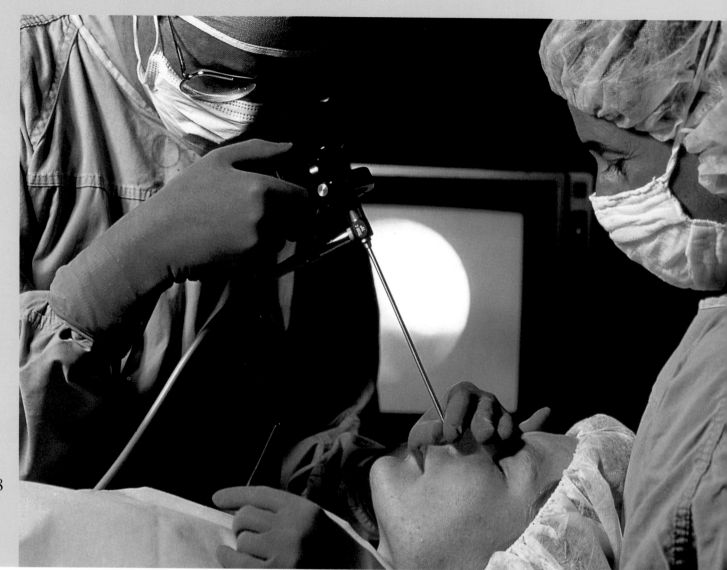

...188

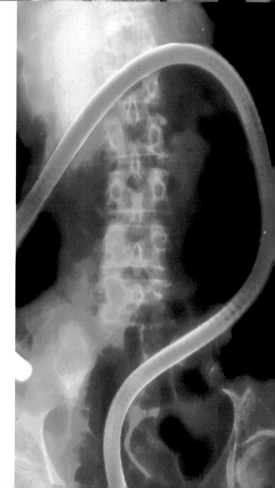

Above: endoscope examination of the nose. The endoscope's field of vision appears on the video monitor in the background.

While doctors become increasingly fascinated with the technology available, there is a sense that many patients are looking for a more holistic approach and that they are beginning to reject the total medicalization of their care.

were regarded as experimental are now commonplace. Total hip replacements for arthritic conditions are now one of the most commonly performed operations in the NHS in Great Britain. The technical advances in surgery have meant a higher survival rate with lower risk of complications.

Childlessness affects 15 per cent of marriages but, in 1978, the work of Patrick Steptoe and Robert Edwards led to the birth of Louise Brown, the first child conceived by in vitro fertilization (IVF) outside the womb. Since then, it has been estimated that two thousand babies have been born by this method. GIFT (gamete introfallopian transfer) is a more recent but less expensive treatment but, as with IVF, success rates vary enormously.

The relatively new advances in keyhole surgery have come about through endoscopy. Endoscopes enable doctors to see inside a body through a fibre-optic telescope and to perform surgical procedures in a minimally evasive way. Endoscopy is most often used as a diagnostic tool to examine the oesophagus, stomach and duodenum. Recent advances have led to hysterectomy and gall bladder removal by endoscope. These techniques mean quicker recovery times and shorter stays in hospital.

Dr Christian Barnard performed the first heart transplant in 1967. Now, the technological advances in anaesthetics and drugs have meant that organs such as the heart, lungs, kidneys, pancreas and even liver can be transplanted from one patient to another and rejection of the new organ is considerably reduced by the use of drugs such as steriods and cyclosporin. It is not now

189...

beyond the realms of possiblity that within the next ten years some operations will be performed by robot, using computer and surgical controls.

In 1953, two Cambridge scientists, James Watson and Francis Crick, published a paper stating that the basic building blocks of life were arranged as a double-helix structure. This mechanism explained how cells could reproduce and led to the science of genetics. Genetic engineering, the science of manipulating genetic material began in 1973, and gene therapy is an area with great potential. Genetic mapping of an individual's chromosomes may identify risks of developing certain inherited diseases. Biologists and geneticists are now experimenting with the insertion of new genes into patients with potentially fatal conditions in the hope that the new gene will proliferate and replace the faulty gene causing the disease. The implantation of specific cells is being used to try and develop a cure for conditions like Parkinson's disease and diabetes.

The pharmaceutical industry is always introducing new drugs to the market. Many of these prove to be versions of already existing drugs, but sometimes a totally new approach to drug therapy is discovered with exciting potential.

All new developments are potentially exciting, but will still carry the same dilemmas for the physician. While doctors become increasingly fascinated with the technology available to help them diagnose and treat patients there is a sense that many patients are looking for a more holistic approach to their care, and that they are beginning to reject the total medicalization of their condition. Doctors have to remain aware that they are ultimately treating the individual and it is the needs of the individual that must be taken into account.

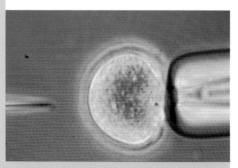

Above: a scientist using a technique known as microinjection to introduce foreign or increased amounts of DNA into the genetic makeup of a cell. The work is done through a light microscope and visualized on a VDU screen. The circular cell is stabilised by a suction tube, right, while the probe introduces the genetic material into the cell. The dark area at the centre of the cell is the nucleus.

Left: a coloured X-ray showing a colonoscope (red), a flexible endoscope, inside a patient's colon.

INDEX

ACKNOWLEDGEMENTS

The publishers would like to thank Dr Paul Downey for his advice and assistance with the chapter on the modern period.

Photographic Acknowledgments: Front cover: Bridgeman/Giraudon.
Ancient Art and Architecture Collection 23 bottom, 24, 27 right, 32 left, 32 top, 34, 35, 82; Frederico Arborio Mella 26, 28, 29, 178 /179, 138 /139; AKG London 6 /7, 9, 40 top right, 40 bottom left, 43, 44 /45, 57, 60 bottom, 69, 71 top, 80, 106, 118 /119, 126 /127, 139, 145, 152 bottom, 170 left, 171, 173. /Academy of Medicine, New York 89 bottom right, 89 bottom left, /Alte Galerie, Landesmuseum Johanneum, Graz 60 /61 top, /Bibliothèque Nationale de France, Paris 48 /49 top, 59, 97, /British Museum 58, /Brussels Library 62 bottom, /Musée du Louvre, Paris 27 left, /Gemäldegalerie, Alte Meister, Dresden 99, /Jefferson Medical College, Philadelphia 136, /Karl-Sudhoff-Institut Collection, Leipzig, University Collection 95, /Kunstmuseum, Basel 66 /67, /Metropolitan Museum of Art, New York 125, /Museu d'Art Catalunya, Barcelona 119, /National Library of Medicine, Bethesda 115, /Österreichische Nationalbibliothek, Vienna 48 /49 bottom, /Palazzo Vecchio, Florence, Studiolo of Grand Duke Francesco I de Medici 85 bottom, /Royal Library, Windsor Castle 73, 74, 75, /Semmelweiss Museum of Medical History, Budapest 112 /113, /Staatsbibliothek, Berlin 4, /Tretyakov Gallery, Moscow 184, /University of Pennsylvania, School of Medicine, Philadelphia 136 /137; AKG London /Erich Lessing 11, 32 /33, /Musée du Louvre, Paris 22, 23 top, /National Museum of Archaeology, Naples 25, /Mauritshuis, The Hague 111, /Museo Ostiense, Ostia 36 /37, /Naturhistorisches Museum, Vienna 8; Bodleian Library 53 bottom, 54 bottom, 54 top, 68 /69; Bridgeman Art Library /British Museum 13, /British Library 53 top, /Cheltenham Art Gallery & Museums, Gloucestershire 96, /Coram Foundation, London 116, 134 /135, /Forbes Magazine Collection, New York 150 /151, /Fratelli Fabbri, Milan 77, 79, /Galleria dell'Accademia, Venice 72, /Giraudon, Paris 5, 44, 98,

Glasgow University Art Gallery 71 bottom, /Guildhall Library, Corporation of London 152 /153, /Lauros-Giraudon 15, /Musée du Louvre, Paris 12, /Prado, Madrid 64 /65, /Private Collection 10/11, 121 bottom, 121 top, /Royal College of Physicians, London 100 /101, /Royal College of Surgeons, London 130 /131, /Royal Holloway & Bedford New College, Surrey 156/157, /University of Bologna Collection 56, 93 right; Jean-Loup Charmet 142; Corbis-Bettmann 3, 144 top, 154, 159, 162 /163, 165, 168 /169, 174, 175, 178; Mary Evans Picture Library endpapers, 4 /5, 20, 42, 62 top, 63, 86, 69 top, 90 /91, 100, 102 /103, 109 bottom, 114 bottom, 117, 122 top, 123, 126, 128 /129, 130, 132 /133, 140 /141, 144 bottom, 146 /147, 147, 150 left, 150 bottom, 157, 160, 161 bottom, 162, 170 right, 180 top, 181 top, 181 bottom, /Sigmund Freud Copyrights 180 left; Hulton Deutsch Collection 78; Istituti Ortopedici Rizzoli in Bologna 122 bottom; Mansell Collection 19, 61 bottom, 76, 112, 143; Reed International Books Ltd 153 right; Réunion des Musées Nationaux /Musée Guimet 17; Royal Botanic Gardens Kew 94; Science Photo Library 30 /31, 90 bottom, 91 top, 107, 128, 141, 154 /155, /Tim Beddow 185 right, 185 left, /Biophoto Associates 148 /149, /Dr Jeremy Burgess 2 /3, 46 /47, 47, 65, 82, 84, 88, 93 left, 104, 105, 109 top, /BSIP, VEM 188 bottom, /Jean-Loup Charmet 66, /GJLP/CNRI 176, /John Greim 188 top, /S Magendra 167, /Prof. Luc Montagnier, Institut Pasteur/CNRI 169 bottom, /Hank Morgan 186, 189, /National Library of Medicine 50, 51 right, 51 left, 85 top, 114 /115, 182, 183, /Philippe Plailly 187, /Rhone-Merieux/CNRI 161 top, /St Mary's Hospital Medical School 169 top, /Alexander Tsiaras 1, 177 left, 177 right; Science & Society Picture Library, Science Museum 36 left, 38 top, 38 bottom, 39 bottom, 39 top, 140, 158; Wellcome Institute Library, London 18 /19, 21, 83, 86 /87, 101 bottom, 110, 120, 124, 132, 164 /165, 172.